Not Too Old for That

Not Too Old for That

How Women Are Changing the Story of Aging

Vicki Larson

ROWMAN & LITTLEFIELD
Lanham • Boulder • New York • London

Published by Rowman & Littlefield
An imprint of The Rowman & Littlefield Publishing Group, Inc.
4501 Forbes Boulevard, Suite 200, Lanham, Maryland 20706
www.rowman.com

86-90 Paul Street, London EC2A 4NE

British Library Cataloguing in Publication Information Available

Library of Congress Cataloging-in-Publication Data

Names: Larson, Vicki, 1956– author.
Title: Not too old for that : how women are changing the story of aging /
    Vicki Larson.
Description: Lanham : Rowman & Littlefield, [2022] | Includes bibliographical
    references and index. | Summary: "The narratives around women at midlife
    and older are more than just sexist and ageist; they're damaging to women's
    physical, emotional, financial, romantic, and sexual health. This book will
    help women break through those tired and hurtful stereotypes to better
    reflect who they are, how they live, and what they want as they age" —
    Provided by publisher.
Identifiers: LCCN 2021047727 (print) | LCCN 2021047728 (ebook) |
    ISBN 9781538155615 (cloth ; alk. paper) | ISBN 9781538155622 (ebook)
Subjects: LCSH: Older women. | Middle aged women. | Aging—Social aspects.
Classification: LCC HQ1061 .L3564 2022 (print) | LCC HQ1061 (ebook) |
    DDC 305.26/2—dc23
LC record available at https://lccn.loc.gov/2021047727
LC ebook record available at https://lccn.loc.gov/2021047728

To Nash and Kit, who have aged me
and kept me young, and to women everywhere

Contents

Foreword

by Wednesday Martin

When I was a younger woman studying anthropology and evolutionary biology, my chosen disciplines had some questions about women. One was *Why do women live past the age of reproduction, since by then they've outlived their reproductive value, and by implication their value, period?* The other was *Why do women and females of other species have orgasms when female orgasm is unnecessary to reproduction?*

These questions—with their implication (or assertion?) that biologically useless women were taking up physical space and climaxing for no reason—got to pass as "neutral scientific inquiry." For many, many years. Imagine the tremendous impact the fact that scientists were basically asking *Why do women who aren't young and nubile even exist?* had on people. I, for one, sat through lectures and read textbooks with a mounting sense of anger that I could not justify. How could I be mad at neutral, irrefutable science?

And yet this science wasn't neutral. Or irrefutable. It was mired in bias, bias that led to the creation and flourishing of theories that not only denigrated women in ways that now seem obvious, but that have since been revisited and found lacking in merit. We now know, for example, that experts from multiple fields concur that female orgasm is at least as functional as it is "extra" . . . and that grandmothers, far from being women who have "outlived their use," have been critical to the flourishing of our species.

We know all this because, thanks to feminism and Title IX, women scientists and social scientists and thinkers have brought new forms of compassion, curiosity, and identification to their endeavors. They've helped correct decades of biased thinking that was warping ideology and science. And limiting women's ability to feel and to be seen and recognized as valuable, vital, sexy, and sexual at all life stages.

Journalist and intersectional feminist cultural critic Vicki Larson continues this important reframing in her book, *Not Too Old for That: How Women are Changing the Story of Aging.* It's a much-needed intervention in our dominant cultural belief—*still*—that postmenopausal women are asexual, invisible, irrelevant, frail, incompetent. That we're dried up, desireless, and undesirable. And that we necessarily face a future of being financially and physically fragile and burdensome to the world to boot.

Larson begins her book by reminding us of an inconvenient and astounding truth: We are fast approaching a watershed moment—2030—when older people will outnumber children for the first time in history. Most of those older people will be *women,* who tend to live longer than men. Older women, in other words, will be the baseline. And she observes that, with many women now living into their nineties, we are not going to spend more than half of our lives being dismissed and diminished, or told to just go away. In fact, not only are we going to challenge the notion that the only good, useful, desirable woman is one in her twenties or thirties, but we are going to disrupt it, redefine it, and own it.

Vicki Larson's brave and much needed blueprint for how to feel and be relevant for your entire life is anchored in an insight about her personal experience. Starting in her late forties, she never felt sexier, more confident, interested or interesting, yet at this very moment, she was being told she was invisible and irrelevant, and being bombarded with products, procedures, and diets that promised her she could buy or buy into "agelessness." What the hell, Larson wants to know, showing the connection between her personal experience, that of most other women, and social justice, is wrong with being a woman who is aging? And why the hell, she wants to know further, wouldn't we do whatever we can to shift received "wisdom" about women and aging that is painting us into a corner of silence, denial, and shame? In chapters on invisibility, menopause, sexuality, sisterhood, money, and limiting gendered scripts about relationships and beauty she does just that: alters our perception of how and who we can be as we age. This is the opposite of "hope in a bottle"—it's radical, meticulously researched, and inspiring possibility in a book.

Acknowledgments

A book that busts the tired and harmful narratives about aging as a woman required me to rely heavily on the work of numerous researchers, authors, and journalists, as well as women who graciously shared with me their own thoughts and experiences. I am incredibly grateful to them and give credit to them not only in the pages of this book, but also in my bibliography.

My entrée into writing books might have happened if Hilary Howard, of the *New York Times,* had not mentioned me to her good friend Sharon Bowers of Miller Bowers Griffin Literary Mgmt. Sharon believed in my first book, which was co-written, enough to become our literary agent, and kept believing in me even when I pitched her numerous off-the-wall book ideas.

I am indebted and full of gratitude to the staff and editors at Rowman & Littlefield and especially to Suzanne Staszak-Silva, who believed there was room for yet another book on midlife and older women.

A huge thank you to all The Lovelies, women I have known for decades, for their kindness, honesty, encouragement, support, shoulders to cry on, and all the years of laughter and friendship. I could not have survived without them. A special thanks to Vincanne Adams, an esteemed scholar, author of numerous books, a sharp and honest critic, and a dear friend who read one of my chapters early on and gave it a thumbs up.

I'm indebted to my late parents, Trude and Bernard, who years ago didn't say, "We told you so," but instead helped me get back on my feet after my first marriage ended, and my late journalism professor, Alan Prince, who helped shape me as a journalist.

Finally, a huge thanks to my children, Nash and Kit, who continue to open my heart every day.

Introduction

The Women We're Becoming

I was forty-five when my thirteen-year marriage imploded, nearly forty-eight when we divorced.

"Why couldn't this have happened ten years ago, when I was younger and prettier?" I remember thinking to myself. "Who will want me now?"

As it turns out, the first man who wanted me was a twenty-six-year-old Brit, a Jude Law look-alike with intense blue eyes, a perfectly chiseled jaw, and a smile that could kill.

It was a mind shift for me. My fifty-five-year-old husband, who had been carrying on a long-term affair with a younger woman—what a cliché!—didn't seem to want me, but a gorgeous younger man did? Maybe this middle-aged thing won't be so bad after all.

It wasn't the only mind shift. I was near the end of my menopausal symptoms, which brought both relief and a sense of dread. What woman hasn't heard the horror stories of menopausal and postmenopausal life? Let's just say it didn't look very promising.

I certainly heard them, but those horror stories never quite materialized. Yes, there were hot flashes and night sweats—there are some real physical changes that can be humbling—but the stereotypes about menopausal women? I did not become unhinged or a bitch (except, of course, when appropriate) or a hormonal moody mess. And that was the other mind shift. All the negative things I heard

1

about aging as a woman that I had bought into and feared? No. Instead I discovered that being alone at midlife with my fertile years behind me led to an inner strength and confidence I didn't realize I had, and a newfound lust for life and, well, lust.

Not to say that it was easy—midlife can feel like a come-to-Jesus moment, when you're suddenly assessing everything in your life, from your fashion style to your hairstyle to your lifestyle. Throw a divorce into midlife, and, well, it's like everything you knew, or thought you knew, is gone and all you're left with is one question: *Now what?*

My "what" turned out to be OK, but not without a few rough spots and bounced checks. Since my divorce at age forty-eight, I became the editor of the lifestyles department at my newspaper; raised two boys into pretty cool young men; had a few long-term romantic relationships and numerous lovers; bought a house; co-wrote a book; traveled and began backpacking and cycling again; nurtured longtime friendships and made new ones; volunteered— in other words, the past decade and a half have been incredibly rich and fulfilling.

And I'm nowhere near done.

Starting in my late forties until today, I have never felt more confident, interested and interesting, vibrant, and juicy—just at the age when I, a postmenopausal woman, am supposed to be asexual, invisible, irrelevant, frail, incompetent.

Excuse me?

I'm just hitting my prime and society is telling me that I'm no longer visible? That I'm undesirable? That I have nothing to offer?

At the risk of sounding a little too full of myself, I was desirable then and still believe I am now, in my mid-sixties. And I am not alone in feeling that way; many older women are enjoying romantic relationships, casual or long-term, with men, women, and non-binary people. More women in their forties and older are having ba-bies—surely they're not all immaculate conceptions! When women like *Facebook* chief operating officer and Lean In founder Sheryl Sandberg are getting engaged at age fifty—and, in her case, to a slightly younger man—I have to question who is telling us that we're invisible and why. And might they be wrong?

Beyond romance and sex, older women are increasingly not invisible. We're running and founding companies; leading coun-tries; appearing on magazine covers, in advertising, and on fashion runways; running in local, state, federal, and presidential elections; winning awards for writing, directing, and starring in movies and TV shows—there even was an older woman cast on the popular reality TV show "The Bachelorette" (although thirty-eight is hardly old).

Yes, we have work to do. Older women still face discrimination in the workplace despite age discrimination laws.[1] We still are under-represented in Hollywood[2] and how we often are represented leaves much to be desired, unless you're OK with being seen as stubborn, unattractive, grumpy, or unfashionable.[3]

Still, there were an unprecedented six women running for president in 2020, ranging in age from thirty-eight to seventy. Clearly, we don't disappear as we age. Clearly, we have plenty to offer. Yet those narratives remain, wreaking havoc on women's physical, emotional, financial, romantic, and sexual health.

Which is how this book came to be.

As much as I felt pretty good about things most of the time at midlife, I also had moments of doubt. I am not immune to the way society talks about "women of a certain age." I also witnessed the decline and death of both my parents in the past decade; was their experience my destiny, too?

I started to look at the many conflicting messages I had been getting about aging as a woman, beyond my inevitable invisibility (and exactly to whom I was going to become the Invisible Woman is unclear). Not just about failing bodies and fleeting beauty, crazy cat ladies and grumpy old ladies (or sweet little old ladies), but also that I'd be dried up, desireless, and undesirable. I'd also be facing a financially and physically fragile and lonely future.

At the same time, I was bombarded with messages about products, procedures, and diets, as well as a bazillion often conflicting articles and books promising me agelessness—or at least the secrets to "aging successfully"—if I just bought them, used them, followed them and whatever new product, procedure, and diet took its place. As if I could buy my way out of aging.

With that kind of relentless messaging, what woman wouldn't dread getting older and perhaps do whatever she could to try to be as "ageless" as she could be for as long as she could?

In truth, those stereotypes are not how many women at midlife and beyond actually feel. How many times have your female friends, relatives, neighbors, and coworkers in their forties, fifties, or older told you that they feel much younger than their age? How many times have you told that to yourself or to others?

Aging, a natural process that's been happening from the second we took our first breath, has been presented to us as something to fear, fight, or deny. Anti-aging creams and diets? If you're against aging isn't that the same as saying you're against living? Fifty is the new forty? What is wrong with fifty being fifty? "You look good for your age?" What is any age "supposed" to look like, and who gets to decide that?

The more I got those messages, the more pissed off I became. I didn't want to fear, fight, or deny aging. It not only seemed counterproductive to living to a healthy old age, but I could also see pretty quickly that if I followed what I was told, it would make me feel pretty crappy about the woman I was and the woman I was becoming—my future self. I was looking for a way to quiet all that noise and be more intentional about how I want to age, what Stanford University psychology professor Laura Carstensen describes as creating a more realistic and kinder vision of a future self[4] and what I might want to do to get there.

Having a more realistic version of our future self matters—it won't serve you, me, or any woman well to live in denial about what might be ahead. And having a kinder version of our future self? Given all the negative messages women have gotten since childhood, this is a no-brainer. If we're talking self-care, that is the ultimate loving thing you can do for yourself.

The negative and ageist perceptions women have about getting older "limit our own choices about how we age," writes AARP's chief executive officer Jo Ann Jenkins in her book, *Disrupt Aging: A Bold New Path to Living Your Best Life at Every Age.*[5]

And they make us feel bad. Proof: my own statement at the beginning of this chapter, "Why couldn't this have happened ten years ago, when I was younger and prettier? Who will want me now?" Why was I so dismissive of the woman I was at the time as well as my future self? (Note to Vicki: You're doing OK. Really.)

Gerontologists have presented the ideas of youthfulness and agefulness as new ways of thinking about aging, one that includes all the experiences that make us who we are and have been becoming.[6]

As cultural critic Vivian Sobchack observes, "every time I try to fixate on a new line or wrinkle, on a graying hair, I try very hard to remember that, on my side of the face in the mirror, I am not so much aging as always becoming."[7]

That sounds so much better than seeking to be ageless, which, as enticing as it sounds, we will never be.

Former first lady Michelle Obama titled her best-selling 2018 memoir *Becoming* for a good reason. "My journey is the journey of always continually evolving," she shares. "There's never a point when you arrive at a thing. . . . If you think there's a point in your life where you stop growing and stop learning, that's sort of sad. Because what else is left?"[8]

Isn't growing older just a continuation of becoming?

Yes, assistant professor of philosophy Hanne Laceulle would say. She rejects the two narratives of aging presented to us—one of decline, which sees getting older as little more than a future of frailty, dependency, loss, and unhappiness; and the more upbeat age-defying narrative, which focuses on remaining youthful, staying productive, and aging well. "Instead of denying or rejecting our vulnerabilities, narratives of becoming suggest that we would do well to face them with an attitude characterized by realism and practical wisdom. This should not only enable us to see what we can do to improve the situation, but also what lies beyond our control and must be gracefully accepted."[9]

As a Boomer, I'm now two decades into trying to reject those ageist narratives, and it's not easy. I'm sorry to say that for Gen X women, who are just entering midlife, those narratives may be hitting them particularly hard. Many Gen Xers married and had children in their thirties and forties, which means midlife is not quite the same for them as it was for my mom's generation, when women wed in their early twenties and were basically an empty-nester in their forties, or for me, whose kids moved out—they did not boomerang back, thankfully—when I was in my fifties, when I needed to help care-give my parents.

"We were an experiment in crafting a high-achieving, more fulfilled, more well-rounded version of the American woman. In midlife, many of us find that the experiment is largely a failure," writes Gen Xer Ada Calhoun in *Why We Can't Sleep: Women's New Midlife Crisis.*[10]

Calhoun observes that her generation was brought up to truly believe that having it all was more than just an option—it was a "mandatory condition" and, inexplicably, totally doable. Whatever Gen X women were doing—forging a career, mothering, being a spouse, finding the illusive sweet work-life spot—they were supposed to excel at it, which, she observes, has only added shame and loneliness to their midlife experience.

Which proves that we gals have been sold a version of what everyone else wants us to be rather than having us decide for ourselves what we want for our future selves. It's time to assess the stories that we have been told about older women, not only in the media, but also among our family, friends, coworkers, and ourselves, and ask how does that impact our lives? In what ways are we marginalized, and in what ways are we helping to contribute to our own marginalization and those of other older women?

There's lots of talk about how midlife can be a time of reinvention, but the pressure to reinvent yourself when you may be caring for aging parents and raising rebellious teens or toddlers while working long hours, or juggling multiple jobs and side hustles just to survive, or reeling from the losses of the coronavirus pandemic, adds another layer of stress and shame—*Oh, I'm supposed to do that, too?*

It's the same with the pressure to look anything other than your actual (translation: old) age.

"There's this incredible denial of middle age going on. It's part of this extended adolescence now going into your forties and fifties. People want to hang onto their youth, so in that sense you're young-young-young 'til you're old,'" says Patricia Cohen, author of *In Our Prime: The Invention of Middle Age.* "I think we're laboring under a different oppressive media image. Before, it was the frigid, asexual, overweight, boring housewife. And now we've gone to 'you have to look like Jennifer Aniston.' If we're not a size-2 figure and have smooth skin from all of this work, then we think we're a failure. We look horrible."[11]

If anything, that means the stereotypes older women are facing aren't going away—they're just shifting and, in some ways, becoming even more onerous.

This is *not* the direction we want to move toward.

What needs to happen, what this book hopes to accomplish, is to help change the narrative about being a woman at midlife and beyond, whether partnered, divorced, widowed or never married; straight or LGBTQ; abled or differently abled; White, Asian, Black, Latina, Indigenous—whatever. To question what we've been told aging would be like and instead ask ourselves, what do we *want* it to be like and how can we get there. To be curious, open-minded, and intentional about the ways we are "becoming."

Why now? Because we are fast approaching a milestone year, 2030, when older people will outnumber children for the first time in history.

And this isn't just a blip. There's a "jaw-dropping global crash in children being born," a July 2020 BBC headline declared,[12] and unless there's some sort of *Handmaid's Tale* dictate—and with the rise of aggressive laws regulating women's reproductive rights in recent years, it has often felt close—it looks like our entire planet will be populated by older people for a long time to come. That has huge ramifications on numerous levels that are clearly outside the scope of this book, but one thing is certain—the vast majority of those people will be women because we tend to live longer than men.

And many of those women will be like me—on their own. Women make up the bulk of the 12.1 million older U.S. adults living alone, according to the Pew Research Center.[13] Women are increasingly remaining single—of the 110.6 million U.S. residents eighteen years and older in 2016 who were single, more than half were women, according to the Census Bureau.[14] Many are divorced. While divorce rates are generally on the decline, there's one age group that's divorcing as if it were the next miracle diet—those aged fifty and older. The number of divorced women sixty-five and older in America has jumped to 14 percent of the population and growing (and women overwhelmingly are the ones seeking divorce).[15] Others are widowed, not only because women live longer than men, but also because women in heterosexual marriages tend to marry men older than they are. According to the 2010 census, there were more than 11 million widows, more than three times the 3 million widowers in the United States.

We women are now living well into our nineties and hundreds; we are not going to spend more than half of our lives being dismissed. In fact, we are going to challenge it, disrupt it, redefine it, and own it.

"I consider myself a proud member of one of the most invisible segments of the population: older women. So, I want to redefine how I live my life in a way that defies what an older woman should look like, talk like, think like, work like, be like and fuck like," says Cindy Gallop, a sixty-something ad executive. "We don't have enough role models in society for women and men that demonstrate you can live your life in a very different way than society expects you to and still be extremely happy."[16]

She is right—we don't have enough role models. But they exist.

Still, if we continue to listen to the outdated narratives of aging as a woman, not only will we harm our present and future selves, but we will also get in our way toward helping to create a less ageist, less sexist, more inclusive future, and that will only trap our daughters into a similar future.

That is why I wrote this book—to help me, and hopefully you, dissect the myth of our invisibility as well as other myths, so we can plan for the next phase of our life. I want to be as intentional as I can be when it comes to my remaining decades—assuming there are, indeed, decades. Like many older women, I am well aware of how truly precious time is.

So, I reached out to the sisterhood of women, talked to numerous experts and disrupters, and culled through studies to absorb as much as I could so I could share what I learned with you. Women today are not going to age as our mothers did—we have many more choices, thankfully. But there are real concerns, too.

To be clear, I am not going to send you on an *Eat, Pray, Love* journey. This book is not about finding yourself, reinventing yourself, or empowering yourself. Women already have power; we just want others to acknowledge it, respect it, encourage it, and nurture and support it. It's also not about yoga retreats, cleanses, daily meditations, intentions, and vision boards—not that there's anything wrong with them.

This book is all about the practicalities of being an older woman today. It's about changing the narrative of who we are, how we live, and what we want.

There is no "right" way to age. So, it's up to each of us to figure out how we want to do that. True, that can seem overwhelming. There are a lot of good books on midlife and aging, some of which I draw from in this book. This also isn't a book about ageism per se, although that is an essential topic that is garnering more attention as the world's population ages. There are already many wonderful books on ageism. This book is a precursor to that discussion because in order to tackle ageism—what has been called the "last acceptable prejudice in America"[17]—we have to check in with ourselves and address our own internalized prejudices about aging, about ourselves, and about the women around us.

Whether we realize or not, we've been perpetuating thoughts and behaviors that make things worse for our aging selves and others.

Once we break that down, we can move past the stereotypes that are holding us back, and rather than feel helpless as the years add up, we can discover and tap into just how much agency we have.

To do that, I am applying two concepts that overlap in their desire to examine and disrupt assumptions and normative practices, spaces, and discourses, and be open to new possibilities—queer and crip theories—to aging.

What does that look like? Take what Alison Kafer, associate professor and chair of Southwestern University's Department of Feminist Studies, writes in her book *Feminist, Queer, Crip*: "How one understands disability in the present determines how one imagines disability in the future; one's assumptions about the experience of disability create one's conception of a better future. If disability is conceptualized as a terrible, unending tragedy, then any future that includes disability can only be a future to avoid."[18]

Now let's swap out "disability" with "aging": "How one understands *aging* in the present determines how one imagines *aging* in the future; one's assumptions about the experience of *aging* create one's conception of a better future. If *aging* is conceptualized as a terrible, unending tragedy, then any future that includes *aging* can only be a future to avoid.

See what I mean?

I'm so done with that.

What we want to do is imagine a better future for ourselves, not one we want to avoid. Before we can do that, though, we first have to confront the bad narratives we've been told and have probably accepted as inevitable.

When people with disabilities "claim crip," turning a word that has long been considered negative into something that many consider positive and empowering, it "can be a way of acknowledging that we all have bodies and minds with shifting abilities," Kafer observes.[19]

And that is exactly what happens as we age.

What makes this book different than other books addressing the intersection of ageism and sexism is that it challenges you to see in what ways you have been influenced by what our culture says you "are" or "should be" as an aging woman, and then guides you to get to where you want to be. Think of this book as a loving big sister or your dearest BFF or a wise elderess who is always there to support you when you need her most.

In chapter 1, we'll delve into the invisibility many women often feel once they hit a certain age while also acknowledging how many marginalized women have always felt invisible in society. Chapter 2 is all about sex, taking on the myth that women become asexual around the time of menopause, with some surprising reasons why women often lose interest in sex (hint: it isn't always about us). Chapter 3 aims an arrow (not necessarily Cupid's) into the heart of our narratives about love, marriage, and romantic relationships, and how the scripts we typically followed in our youth don't always work for what we're seeking in our later years. In chapter 4, we explore the quest for "ageless" beauty at any cost and highlight ways some women come to accept and embrace their aging bodies. Chapter 5 is all about busting the myth of the mean girl/mean woman, and the growing importance of female friendship and chosen families. Chapter 6 puts health and menopause and the stereotypes of frailty and dependency on the exam table, and in chapter 7 we'll spend time on finances. The final chapter aims to find ways we ourselves can be the loving big sister, dearest BFF, or wise elderess for other women.

I began this journey as a way to figure out my own life. As I began to work my way through the BS messages—and I am so tired of the BS—and to consider the possibilities, I realized that I probably wasn't the only older woman seeking ways to ignore the noise of what others perceive us to be so we can just get on with living our best life. And if there's one thing we gals do best, it's making sure that we uplift the sisterhood and do it together.

Shall we start?

1

The Amazing
Invisible Woman

A woman who goes through life without taking any notice of society's perception of her becomes the most feared individual on the planet. This is because patriarchy wants to reduce her to an insecure, submissive female and as long as she rejects the notion of validation, she is perceived as a threat to the status quo.

—British writer Mohadesa Najumi[1]

You can't see me, you can't stop me.

—Frankie Bergstein, *Grace and Frankie*[2]

I was never sure when I was supposed to become invisible. For many years, I didn't even know that was where I was headed.

And then one day, the media blared it.

"It's official: many women become invisible after 49" was the *Reuters* headline on April 13, 2015, a day that will clearly live in female infamy.[3]

Reuters wasn't just talking about women's invisibility in terms of no longer being able to attract the "male gaze." Actually, what the news agency spoke to was much worse and with much broader implications: how middle-aged and older women were being excluded from the conversation—*any* conversation.

"In a world of data-driven policies, there is one group in society that barely registers and is at risk of missing out on crucial resources and services, according to researchers—older women. Much international data, including metrics on health, employment, assets, and domestic violence, appears to back up the anecdotal view that women become invisible in middle age. The data sets start at the age of fifteen and stop abruptly at forty-nine. Experts said the limited age framework stems from a focus on women of reproductive age, assumptions about the limited economic role of older women, and age discrimination that overlooks sexuality and violence in older women's lives."

There's so much in there to process that I almost did the stereotypical older woman thing—pour myself a generous glass of wine and snuggle with my numerous cats and a pint of Ben & Jerry's. I don't have any cats—not that there's anything wrong with them—just a rescue dog, but I would certainly adopt however many cats I needed just to have researchers see that I, along with the nearly quarter of the world's population of women who are beyond the age of popping out babies, still have value.

Is a woman's reproductive age the only thing that matters? Is that what makes us invisible and irrelevant?

When we talk about the invisibility of older women, we often aren't on the same page. There are so many first-person essays of "the moment I became invisible" that it's hard to know if there's a universal moment—we just "know," or accept, that it's inevitable. (I have yet to read a first-person essay by a middle-aged man about the moment that he felt invisible. Not to say that they don't feel that way; it's just that no one expects them to.)

For some women, "invisibility" means the loss of the male gaze. For some, it's about the general loss of being seen as desirable. For some, it's about being dissed by younger people (including younger women). For some, it's about employment discrimination. For some, it's about ableism. For some, it's about racism. For some it's about discrimination on all the levels, full stop.

What is it that makes a woman become invisible? Is it truly our reproductive age? In her 2012 book *In Our Prime: The Invention of Middle Age,* journalist Patricia Cohen pretty much says yes.

NO BABIES? SORRY, BABY

As the title reveals, middle age is an invented concept "pulled along by age-graded institutions, industrialization, and urbanization, as well as drops in birth and mortality rates" right around the turn of the twentieth century. The term "geriatrics"—hardly a term any woman in her right mind would want to embrace—was coined around the same time.[4] But what truly helped propel the invention of midlife was the fact that more women were having fewer children, she says.

You can see how some people might turn that fact around and blame us for our own plight.

There was no concept of midlife until 1895, when the word was included in a dictionary, Funk & Wagnalls, for the first time, defined as "the part of life between youth and old age."[5]

But oh, what happened in that part of life! For women, it typically involved a lot of having babies and mothering. In 1800, Cohen writes, most women had around seven children and spent a good seventeen years of their life either pregnant or breastfeeding—seventeen years!—after which they were, quite understandably, pretty weakened or disabled. "By the time all her children were grown, she was well into her sixth decade—or more likely dead," Cohen writes.[6]

Fast forward a hundred years and now women are having just two or three children. By the time their kids left home, they were around fifty-three years old, giving them nearly two good decades of freedom until they died, typically around age seventy-one. "Adulthood was no longer an unvarying, seamless whole filled with farmwork and childrearing until death. Middle-aged women were able for the first time to turn to other pursuits, like fashion, shopping, working, and volunteering. There was life after children."[7]

Here's to life after children! My gal friends and I, all in our sixties, have been absolutely enjoying that life. But the bigger picture at the time meant that at midlife, a woman could no longer have children, and if she was no longer breastfeeding and mommying, well, who was she and what, exactly, was her purpose? Did she even have a purpose anymore?

Never mind if women didn't have children, either because they didn't want them (a rarity in those days) or couldn't have them. Sadly, that didn't spare them from midlife stereotypes. "If middle-aged women were devalued, it was because society constricted their options," Cohen writes. "Primarily typecast as mothers and housewives, in society's view they became functionally unnecessary after menopause and after their children grew up."

"Functionally unnecessary" sounds unnecessarily harsh. Surely, they were still loved and wanted by their spouse, children, friends, and relatives. But even as late as 1969, women weren't faring much better. As *Everything You Ever Wanted to Know About Sex* (*But Were Afraid to Ask)* informed us, "To many women, the menopause marks the end of their useful life. They see it as the onset of old age, the beginning of the end. Having outlived their ovaries, they think they may have outlived their usefulness as human beings. They may fear that the remaining years will just be marking time until they follow their glands into oblivion."[8]

The end of our useful life? Following our glands into oblivion? Who would even think that, let alone write something like that and expect anyone to buy it? Except the book was the No. 1 best-selling book around the world and had millions of readers. (A 1972 movie of the same name made by Woody Allen and loosely based on the book grossed more than $18 million in North America alone, so there's that.)[9]

No surprise it was written by a man—Dr. David Reuben. (For the record, Reuben, who had angered feminists and gays for his views in this book and ones that followed, had questionable professional credentials and relied on scant academic references and eventually had to escape to Costa Rica, but not before causing a lot of grief for women because of his views.)[10]

No surprise either that it was published during the decade of the sexual revolution, just a few years after the "Pill" was approved for contraceptive use in 1960, which gave women the freedom to decide if and when to have children independent of a spouse or romantic partner,[11] and coming at the beginning of the second wave of feminism.[12]

In other words, it was a period when women had power to control the trajectory of their own life. They had other choices besides just having children and being mothers.

Imagine turning to *Everything You Ever Wanted to Know About Sex* (*But Were Afraid to Ask)* for help, as millions did, only to be told you have used up your usefulness, or your wife is about to? How many women, and men, believed that to be true? How might that impact their views and actions? (My parents actually had a copy of it on a bookshelf in their bedroom, where all the "sexy" books were, and I hope they didn't take that crap to heart.)

This is why the old narratives about aging as a woman are dangerous—someone says it, she believes it, he believes it, they believe it, and before you know it, it is seen as "natural" for all women. But those narratives date back to a time when a woman's place was in the home, whether she wanted to be there or not, and when motherhood was her main role along with being a wife.

The idea that women are only "useful" if they can pop out babies is a troublesome one, and one that has little to do with how women live today. It's also a socially constructed view, and rather misogynistic because it centers on what men want.

As OB-GYN Dr. Jen Gunter writes in *The Menopause Manifesto,* "it's misogynistic to tie a description for one-third or possibly one-half of a woman's life to the function of her uterus and ovaries."[13] Just imagine trying to define a man's life by how well his penis is functioning or the quality of his sperm. Not going to happen.

Honestly, no woman I know thinks or acts like she's useless just because she's no longer fertile. While some women may feel some temporary sadness about that—and for others, great relief—many more women at midlife and older experience what American anthropologist Margaret Mead called "postmenopausal zest."

In a 1959 *Life* magazine article, Mead bemoaned the fact that society spends way too much time focusing on the brief period when a woman is raising young children—and it is brief in the course of a lifetime—and not the many fruitful decades ahead of her.

"Motherhood is like being a crack tennis player or ballet dancer—it lasts just so long, then it's over," she said. "We've made an abortive effort to turn women into people. We've sent them to school and put them in slacks. But we've focused on wifehood and reproductivity with no clue about what to do with mother after the children have left home. We've found no way of using the resources of women in the 25 years of post-menopausal zest."[14]

Women themselves, however, saw things differently. In fact, they felt that zest and were eagerly acting on it.

"A SECOND YOUTH"

"Menopause" didn't appear in English-language dictionaries until the late 1880s although the term had been around since 1821, according to Susanne Schmidt's 2020 book *Midlife Crisis: The Feminist Origins of a Chauvinist Cliché,*[15] and it became a medical category shortly thereafter. Because those involved in medicine were men at the time—Elizabeth Blackwell, America's first female doctor, received her medical degree in 1850; a century later, the percentage of female doctors was barely 6 percent—let's just say that they were not kind to women at this stage of their life. In fact, they considered menopause to be "an illness in need of treatment or an indication of a body in disorder"[16] instead of a normal condition like, say, puberty.

Meanwhile, feminists at the time, such as educator, minister, and suffragist leader Anna Garlin Spencer, saw menopause for what it was—"a second youth,"[17] when women were finally free of their domestic duties and could become "a citizen of the world." In other words, women felt liberated no matter what the male doctors were saying.

Clearly women have been feeling that postmenopausal zest for centuries. So why are we sold a different narrative, even today? Historian Susan Mattern doesn't beat around the bush explaining why. The medicalization and pathologizing of menopause into a "syndrome" was a way to weaken women when our power is rising, she suggests in her book, *The Slow Moon Climbs: The Science, History, and Meaning of Menopause*, as it was in Spencer's day and as it is now. "Dominant groups can be very creative in inventing new ways of oppressing people," she writes.[18]

Imagine if menopause was viewed as a natural event that was purposely designed for a reason, most likely one that made evolutionary sense, such as the "grandmother hypothesis," which emphasizes the importance of non-reproductive women to human survival. How would women feel about it and midlife? But, instead menopause "came to be seen as a deficiency of the chemical estrogen, which in turn came to be seen as the essence of femininity," she writes.

Isn't it funny how we don't talk about testosterone as being the essence of masculinity?

Menopause was seen as a disease, and not just any old disease but the "worst" kind—one that automatically made women undesirable to men.[19]

The way we talk about menopause and female aging even today comes down to what Mattern believes is an "age-specific backlash against the challenge women pose to men as sex roles become less differentiated."[20]

In other words, older women who come into their own and display their postmenopausal zest are a threat. To men.

Gail Sheehy battled the idea of women outliving their usefulness in her groundbreaking 1976 book *Passages,* offering women (mostly White, well-educated women on the East and West coasts) the promise of opportunities once they hit midlife. She saw middle age as a time when women could reappraise their lives post-children and even bust free from traditional gender roles in their hetero marriages. Her message was met, as Schmidt details, with a misogynist backlash.

All of which reinforced the idea that women become invisible and irrelevant at midlife. Can't pop out babies anymore? Outlived your ovaries? Well, guess what gals—we're useless. Even though about 20 percent to 25 percent of Boomers don't have kids, either by choice or chance. For Gen Xers, it's about 40 percent.[21] And with the existential crisis of climate change hanging over us, more Millennials and other women of childbearing age are questioning whether to have children at all.[22]

Prizewinning Danish author Dorthe Nors knows the future of those women well. She not only writes novels about childfree, middle-aged single women, on "the brink of disappearing—or you could say—on the brink of losing their license to live," but she also is one. "If a woman has kids, she will always be a mother, but a woman who has chosen not to procreate and who now no longer is young and sexy is perceived by many as a pointless being. . . . A middle-aged woman who's not preoccupied with handling herself or taking care of someone else is a dangerous, erratic being. What is she up to? And what's the point of her being up to anything? She has no children, she has no family, the only thing she has is her own life."[23]

God forbid a woman has her own life!

Gen X mothers entering midlife now are most likely going to have to wait to tap into that postmenopausal zest. In the 1950s, '60s, and '70s, women were around twenty years old when they married; in 2020, the median age was twenty-eight, according to the U.S. Census.[24] In 2016, college-educated women were around thirty-one years old when they became mothers for the first time.[25] Even if they stop at one child—and women are increasingly having only children[26]—their kids will still be young around the time they allegedly become invisible.

One thing Gen X women have going for them along with Boomers is that more of them have been or still are in the workplace, giving them other identities than just "wife" and "mom"—if they even are a wife or a mom. This matters because the more roles a woman has that aren't related to fertility and childbearing, the more positive they generally feel about aging.[27]

This new middle age, ages forty-five to sixty-five, has been called "middlescence" by gerontologist Barbara Waxman. "Think of it like a second adolescence. We have questions about our place in the world and are wondering about our future. Our sense of self and identity is evolving. Just like adolescence, Middlescence is emerging from a demographic and cultural shift in our country, and naming it will change the way we experience this impactful part of our lives."[28]

NEVER-ENDING FERTILITY?

Still, this is what women have been constrained by—the idea that we are only desirable and visible if we are fertile, and fertility has a limited window. Except it doesn't anymore. In 2019, a seventy-three year-old Indian woman gave birth to twins via in vitro fertilization (IVF).[29] In 2021, a fifty-seven-year-old New Hampshire woman gave birth to a son via IVF.[30] In 2018, the Buck Institute in Marin County, north of San Francisco, was gifted $6 million to create a Center for Female Reproductive Longevity and Equality to develop strategies to prevent or delay ovarian aging, and that has since received billions more. The money came from philanthropist Nicole Shanahan and her husband, Google co-founder Sergey Brin. Shanahan had problems getting pregnant, and wondered, why do women have to suffer?

"Ten percent of women are infertile by the time they turn 35, and just five years later at the age of 40, a woman has only a 5 percent chance of becoming pregnant. I committed myself to help future generations of women have more choices," she said. "Personally, I find it crazy that my reproductive organs are considered geriatric long before any other organ even begins to show the slightest decline. I find it even crazier that we have conceded to this narrative for half of the human species."[31]

No matter how you feel about women having babies into their forties, fifties, and sixties—even seventies—or whether you would want that for yourself, if science is truly able to prevent or delay ovarian aging, and women can have healthy babies way beyond age thirty-five, aka "geriatric pregnancy" or "advanced maternal age," it does beg the question: how can anyone continue to justify using fertility as the marker of a woman's visibility, attractiveness, and "usefulness"?

Researchers Shirley Chan, Alyssa Gomes, and Rama Singh say we shouldn't. In a paper they authored in 2020, they argue that delayed marriage and reproduction is having a huge impact on menopause. It's evolving. "We propose a *shifting mate choice-shifting menopause* model which posits that, as the age of mate choice/marriage shifts to older ages, so will the age at menopause, and that menopause is a transient phase of female fertility; it can de-evolve, be delayed, if not disappear completely," they write (researchers' emphasis).[32]

Not immediately, but over time.

This is a game changer for how women experience midlife and how society views middle-aged women. All the horror stories women hear about midlife, menopause, and invisibility would disappear, simply because they can have babies at any age they want, if they want them, just like men.

It's also incredibly unfair that all women, some of whom don't even want to have babies or who can't have babies, are being judged for their fertility anyway.

Yet that narrative, that women become invisible at midlife, is a hard one to bust through. Because there are many ways women experience themselves becoming invisible. They no longer experience the male gaze—sometimes for better, actually. They're ignored by baristas, wait staff, bartenders, the front-desk clerk at the gym. They are passed over for promotions at work or aren't offered interviews for positions even though they are qualified. And they don't see their lives portrayed accurately, if at all, in TV shows and movies.

As has been well documented, Hollywood has few uses for women past a certain age—just 21.4 percent of characters over age forty were female in all the films released in 2014,[33] and in 2019, there were no women over age fifty cast in a leading role. Not one.[34] And the few older women who are featured, as was mentioned in the Introduction, are overwhelmingly portrayed as stubborn, unattractive, grumpy, and unfashionable.

Of course, we don't expect Hollywood to be "real" life. It's fantasy and we understand that at a certain level. But for whatever reason, our celebrity- and reality-TV-obsessed culture has us increasingly looking to media stars as our role models on how to age.

This is probably not a good idea.

So much about female celebrities is based on their looks, or more accurately, fading looks, and the need to do whatever it takes to stay youthful looking (more about this in chapter 4). It would be one thing if it were just men who were selling women on that. All too often, however, we women are our own worst enemies, because we've taken that message and internalized it.

The past few years have seen more middle-aged and older female celebrities featured in ads and on catwalks and magazine covers. When Jennifer Lopez, at age fifty, strutted the Versace catwalk in 2019 wearing the same vibrant green and deeply plunging dress she wore to the Grammys two decades earlier, *Guardian* associate fashion editor Jess Cartner-Morley was mixed. As much as she felt like she was "cheering for my team" in seeing a vibrant older woman owning her power, the forty-something Cartner-Morley wondered about the message the suddenly visible invisible women were sending. "[T]he modern rebranding of 50 is really all about the visual element: the smooth skin, taut abs, being able to wear the same revealing dress you wore two decades earlier."[35]

In other words, the only way to be visible as a middle-aged and older woman nowadays is to, once again, rely on our looks.

Ugh. How can this possibly work to our benefit?

MORE THAN YOUTH

The "official" age of a woman's invisibility may be forty-nine, but some women say they experience it much earlier than that. That was former supermodel Paulina Porizkova's experience once she turned forty years old, and she was vocal about it.[36] Once she hit her fifties, things, perhaps not surprisingly, didn't seem to get better.[37] "Being a woman today—and throughout thousands of years—has taught us that societal expectations of women are, primarily, to be pretty. It has also taught us that older women are invisible and of very little value."

(Porizkova and screenwriter and producer Alan Sorkin went to the 2021 Academy Awards together, a second date, so I'm not sure she's quite as invisible as she says she is.)

As she approached her fiftieth birthday, author Ayelet Waldman made a similar confession to a friend: "I'm turning 50. Then that's it. I become invisible. . . . I had no idea that as soon as I got to this

age, to be a 50-year-old woman, the sexism gets completely complicated by this idea that not only are you incompetent as a woman,
but you're incompetent because you've reached your senescence!
Or something."[38]

For women like Porizkova, whose livelihood was based on her
beauty and youth, it may be somewhat understandable that wrinkles and sags might make them feel unseen, unappreciated, and
perhaps unemployed (still, she looks amazing). But why would a
woman like Waldman, whose livelihood has nothing whatsoever to
do with her looks—not that she's not attractive; she is—but is based
on her wits and writing talent feel as if she's become invisible? Her
novels and essays don't seem to scream, I'm old!

"The sad thing about watching yourself becoming invisible is
you can start to believe it," writes former advertising executive Jane
Evans on her website for "The Uninvisibility Project," which she
founded in 2019 to highlight the stories of midlife women. "It's hard
to value yourself when your industry doesn't want your wisdom
and experience and it's even harder to keep going when society
doesn't value you full stop."[39]

I know that feeling intimately. When my newspaper needed to
find ways to cut costs, it offered buyouts, but only to those past age
sixty who had been with the paper for at least twenty years—in other
words, those who were making the most money, true, (FYI, print
journalism is not a highly paid profession) but also those who had a
depth and breadth of knowledge that could not easily be replaced.

That said, society has long neglected, dismissed, or outright ignored the experiences of many marginalized women—queer, trans,
larger-sized, disabled, single, and childfree and childless women—
who have felt invisible before they even became middle-aged.

There are lessons to be learned from that, but it's no one's
responsibility to provide "invisibility inspiration" for anyone.
Marginalized women have many more challenges on so many levels
and face much more discrimination than women who have not been
marginalized (besides the reality of being a woman), but suddenly
are confronted with invisibility simply because they've gotten older.

While lesbian and bisexual women don't seem to be quite as
concerned about changes to their attractiveness and fertility at
midlife as hetero women do,[40] they all too often find themselves
becoming a triply invisible minority—a woman, a gay woman, and
an old woman.[41]

THE GREAT EQUALIZER

When it comes to invisibility, disability appears to be the great equalizer. "Sooner or later, if we live long enough . . . we will all become disabled," queer disability studies expert Robert McRuer argues.[42]

Some stats: There are an estimated 61 million people in the United States living with a disability. Many are African Americans—29 percent versus 20 percent who are White—and many are women. Some 27 million American women live with a disability—whether their limitations are sensory, cognitive, self-care, or ambulatory or mobility—and a full 50 percent of women over the age of sixty-five have at least one disability, according to the Centers for Disease Control.[43]

Ola Ojewumi is one. Diagnosed with a heart condition as a child that led to a heart and kidney transplant, she has limited mobility— she relies on a wheelchair—and a chronic illness.

"For years, I despised being disabled. . . . But eventually, I got tired of concealing my existence as a black woman with a disability. The world was already doing that for me," writes Ojewumi, founder of an educational nonprofit, in an essay titled "I'm Celebrating My Disabled Black Girl Magic Because I'm Done Feeling Invisible."[44] "Black women living with disabilities deal with the triple-headed monster of racism, sexism, and ableism. I've recognized that I will have to work exponentially harder than most other people to achieve my goals. I've faced judgment on every front, but I use that to my advantage. Most people underestimate wheelchair users, women, and people of color. So, I boss up, put my wheelchair in drive, and prove them wrong, playing on their ignorance as I climb the ladder to success."

Ojewumi, in her late twenties, is already feeling invisible. Growing older is a gift for someone with a disability, she tells me, but a scary gift, as aging often adds disabilities atop of disabilities.[45] (We'll explore that further in chapter 6.)

All the "isms" are keeping women from fully being who we are, and how we want and deserve to be fully seen.

The intersection of ableism, sexism, and racism—what has been called "intersectional invisibility"[46]—makes for a particularly onerous form of oppression, one that further marginalizes people within marginalized groups. Adding ageism into the mix, or homophobia, takes invisibility to another level.

So does adding a women's status as a mother—or not.

Even if women are no longer fertile, our role as a mother still matters. According to the Centre for Ageing Better, a U.K. nonprofit, "older people are commonly referred to with their role within the family rather than as an individual, with older women ('gran', 'grandmother') often featuring in the role of the carer."[47] The only way to "see" older women is in relation to what we are doing for others.

That's why women who age without children, especially if they're unpartnered, feel invisible and marginalized by a society that's family-centric, notes Kirsty Woodard, an advocate for child-less people and founder of the UK-based Ageing Well Without Children.[48]

They also age faster, notes Tel Aviv University lecturer Kinneret Lahad in her book, *A Table for One: A Critical Reading of Singlehood, Gender and Time*. Not literally, of course. But there's no other way to explain how thirty-something single women are considered old—and thus invisible—while thirty-something married moms are considered "young mothers."[49]

CREATING DIGITAL IDENTITIES

If women are going to flip the narrative about becoming invisible at a certain age, one way to do that is to consider that another world is possible, as crip theory scholar Robert McRuer would say.[50]

Many are creating that world online, flying in the face of the belief that women past a certain age are "technology inept and digitally illiterate."[51]

No, we are not. In fact, women, especially Black women, tend to use social media more than men and White people "to create, curate and build congruent and integral layers of 'best self' identity."[52]

It's been particularly important for queer and trans Black women—women who often face marginalization within their own marginal-ized communities—according to Northeastern University assistant professor Moya Bailey. In her 2021 book *Misogynoir Transformed*, Bailey details how they are addressing anti-Black misogyny, which she calls misogynoir, by creating digital communities to change the narrative about their lives and as a way to "reduce harm."[53]

In a mom-centric world, older childfree and childless women are finding support and community online, too, at places like Gateway Women, a global organization providing resources for involuntarily childless women, especially to plan for aging, and The NotMom. In fact, midlife and older women have increasingly been turning to social media to construct more positive, playful, and sometimes provocative identities as they age.

"Whereas most existing scholarship on visual depictions of age focuses on images that are controlled by other people (e.g., advertisers, community groups), I show how #over50 lifestyle Instagrammers and bloggers control their self-representations," writes Dr. Laura McGrath in her study of women aged fifty to seventy who have turned to Instagram and blogs to not only make themselves visible, but to also connect with other older women to create a supportive community, inspire each other, and offer positive perceptions of aging as a woman.[54]

"As with all literate practices, these women's self-representations—their multimodal performances of identity—mean and do something within a complex web of social practices, discourses on age and gender, offline experiences and relationships, professional goals, personal needs and aspirations, cultural values and assumptions, mediating technologies, and so forth. All of these influences are at work as midlife and older women engage digital literacies in the service of self-expression, inspiration, connection, and promotion."

For Alessandra Bruni Lopez y Royo, becoming a professional model at age forty-six after a career as an academic was a way to strip away some of the invisibility she felt growing older.[55] Now in her sixties, Alex B.—her modeling name—encourages older women to model, too, if not for a career, then at least to share their images on Instagram and other social media sites to challenge and subvert society's narrow version of beauty and damaging stereotypes of aging female bodies. Images are powerful.

So are words. There's a greeting that South Africa's Zulu tribe members say to each other —"Sawubona," which translates into "I see you, you are important to me, and I value you."[56] What a kind and loving way to acknowledge another person, to let them know that they're not invisible, that they are accepted for all that they are.

Aging women deserve to be valued, accepted, and seen, not just online.

Still, invisibility can be a type of liberation for women, essayist and *How to Disappear* author Akiko Busch argues, allowing us to tap into our authentic self by letting go of a need to constantly be seen.[57] Like Harry Potter's invisibility cloak, there's much to be said about having a secret power.

THINGS TO THINK ABOUT

In what ways have you felt invisible?
In what ways have others been invisible to you?
In what ways and in what situations do you want to be seen?
In what ways do you make yourself seen?
In what ways has your invisibility been beneficial?

2

"I'll Have What She's Having"

Women were not allowed to have passion at sixty. We were supposed to become grandmothers and retreat into serene sexlessness.

—Erica Jong, *Fear of Dying*[1]

On a trip to see her mother in Florida a few years ago, my friend Eve was confused. Her mom was acting really odd.

"I need to confide in you," her mother finally said, in hushed tones that could not conceal her giddiness. "I've been seeing a man."

OK, Eve thought to herself, relieved it wasn't something health-related or that she'd wired money to a Nigerian prince. Still, that didn't explain her unusual behavior.

Then her mother said something Eve did not expect to hear.

"Evie, Evie, how'd he know what to do with his fingers? Has that ever happened to you?"

What "happened" was that Eve's mother had experienced her first orgasm. She was ninety-one.

All of Eve's gal-pals and I screamed with joy when she later shared that story with us. Eve's mother was a Holocaust survivor, a widow after fifty years of marriage to Eve's father, who Eve was pretty sure was a closeted gay man. After decades of no-doubt unfulfilling sex, Eve's mom finally got to experience the sexual pleasure she deserved, and—no surprise—she wanted more. But by that time, her "handy" lover had moved on to other women in her retirement community

Like some women at midlife, Eve's mom was more than happy to give up on whatever sex she and Eve's father were having when she was postmenopausal. They had two beautiful children, whom she adored, and that's all that really mattered. Her own pleasure did not. Until it did.

I think of Eve's mother's story whenever I hear people—usually men, but not always—say that middle-aged and older women aren't interested in sex. OK, maybe some aren't. But imagine if Eve's mom had been having orgasmic sex all her life, or at least some of her life. Sure, she may have lost interest in sex for a while when her kids were young or when she was going through menopause or when the stresses of life were too exhausting and all she wanted to do was watch *The Crown* reruns or read a book.

Sexual desire isn't static.[2] In fact, it's quite fluid—there's no "linear decline" over time, according to Dr. Bianca Fileborn of the University of Melbourne, but more like "something that ebbs and flows across the life span."[3]

Right, sexual desire ebbs and flows for women of all ages and men as well. But you wouldn't necessarily know that from the narratives about hetero women. Here's what we hear—that we're dried up, lack desire, aren't capable of having sex, and even if we wanted sex and were able to have it, we wouldn't be able to attract someone who'd want to have sex with us anyway. And on the rare occasions that a middle-aged woman does spark a man's interest, then she's a cougar if he's younger and a gold digger if he's older. Meanwhile, lesbian women are supposedly doomed to live with "lesbian bed death" as they age.

None of that is true, of course, but people tend to cling to their outdated beliefs about women's sexuality because it's easier than accepting that women are as sexual as men are and aren't even well-suited for monogamy.

Imagine what it would be like if women approached their middle and older years knowing that their sexual desires and desirability ebbed and flowed, and that those fluctuations were perfectly "normal." What if women approached their middle and older years knowing that a desire for passion, pleasure, and intimacy doesn't go away as you age and can, in fact, increase and even take on new forms? Would we make different choices in deciding with whom, how, when, and in what way we have sex? Would we be more accepting of ourselves as sexual beings? Would we demand better sex and more pleasure from our partners? Would we enjoy sex more? And would we be better able to talk openly about our sexual concerns with our health care providers?

IT'S NOT YOU, IT'S HIM

Last year, a slightly older man I connected with on a dating website let me know early in our messaging that he was concerned that a woman my age might have lost her libido. He did, however, let me know that, at age sixty-seven, his equipment, is "very good" — or so he had been told.

When he wrote that to me, I couldn't help but think of the classic scene in *When Harry Met Sally*, in which Sally, played by Meg Ryan, loudly and convincingly fakes an orgasm for Harry, played by Billy Crystal, while they're eating in a deli. When a wait staffer comes by to take an order from an older woman seated nearby, the woman says, "I'll have what she's having."

(For the record, most women do not orgasm through penis-vagina penetration; just ask Eve's mom and every sex educator who has ever written an article or book, given a TEDx talk or lecture, been interviewed, or counseled a struggling couple.)

In truth, I haven't been sexual with a man that old, but I've been with men a lot younger than he is and whose equipment was not "very good" or even "good." In fact, studies indicate that erectile dysfunction is on the rise in men younger than forty.[4] Other studies indicate men aged fifty to fifty-nine are more than three times as likely to have trouble getting and maintaining an erection, and have less of an interest in sex compared with men aged eighteen to twenty-nine.[5] Erectile dysfunction is more likely to happen to men in poor physical and emotional health, which most certainly many men have experienced from the global pandemic and economic meltdown. And having COVID-19 may create its own ED problems, research has found.[6]

But that's not the narrative we hear. All we hear is that older women are the ones who lose interest in sex or are dried up, and older men are always good to go—a myth that actually hurts men and wreaks havoc on the relationships they have with the women who love them, according to sex researcher Sarah Hunter Murray.

"Study after study continues to suggest that men's and women's sexual desire is more similar than different," she writes.[7]

Not all older women lose interest in sex, although some do. It could be that many of those women never had a big interest in sex anyway, even when they were younger, or that they never experienced good sex (hello, Eve's mom), or have had sexual trauma, or have health issues that make penetration painful. For some women, sex with the same person year after year may just be boring. And for others, they are basically forced into sexual abstinence because they either lack a sexual partner or have a partner who can no longer be sexual or doesn't want to be.

That happens more than you might think. "Contrary to the misperception that women are usually in control of determining whether an older heterosexual couple ceases sexual activity, sexual desire more commonly declines among men, usually due to erectile dysfunction," note clinical psychologist Dr. Michelle Maciel and psychologist Luciana Laganà.[8] "The stereotype of the asexual menopausal woman could originate mainly from the sexual functioning problems of aging men, which are not conducive to older women's expression of sexual interest."

Again, that is not what we generally hear when people talk about menopausal and postmenopausal women losing desire.

Of course, there's more to a man than his penis when it comes to sex, but if his penis is tripping him up, what's a horny older woman to do?

Maybe pay for sex.

SEARCHING FOR PLEASURE

In Sophie Hyde's movie *Good Luck to You, Leo Grande,* which began filming in 2021, Emma Thompson plays a fifty-five-year-old sexually inexperienced widow who hires a sex worker in his early twenties. Her character, Nancy Stokes, is looking for adventure, connection, and sex. Not just any sex, but really good sex. Almost six decades into her life, she's never experienced it.[9]

According to the plotline, while her late husband gave her a wonderful home and a wonderful family, wonderful sex was not part of their life together. "There are nuns with more sexual experience than me," Thompson's character says. So she hires a much younger sex worker for a night of bliss.

While the movie is, well, just a movie, it presents an interesting concept—if older women can't find romantic partners around their age to date, couple with, or marry, or if they aren't interested in a full-time romantic partner at all, just some good sex, why must they be forced into sexual celibacy? Why not hire a sex worker for a night, or several nights, of bliss? And why not pick a much younger one?

Although women who pay for sex is still a tiny fraction compared to men, women, both single and partnered, increasingly have been seeing that as an option and a number are traveling to places in the Caribbean or Gambia or Thailand for what's alternately called "sex tourism" or "romance tourism."[10] It's also given rise to straight male escort services like Cowboys4Angels, featured in Showtime's hit series *Gigolos* and, according to its founder Garren James, brought in nearly $2 million in 2014.[11]

In one admittedly small study, twenty-one Australian women aged eighteen to sixty-nine explained why they paid for sex: for therapy, such as helping them with medical and trauma issues; to learn, whether it's different types of sex play or new sexual experiences like a threesome, or to explore their sexual orientation; and for intimacy, such as touch and affirmations. But they overwhelmingly said it was for pleasure—their own pleasure, not the man's.[12]

They found that taking care of their needs without "feeling obliged to give sex in ways that men might expect of them," as one might have to do with a romantic partner or even in a hookup, was both liberating and empowering.

It's pretty rare for women to have such one-sided sexual experiences, especially in a culture that does not place much emphasis on women's sexual pleasure. And given how few hetero women are having orgasms with their romantic partners—according to a 2018 study, heterosexual women are behind every other group happily getting off, including lesbians and bisexual women, and hetero, bisexual, and gay men—we are missing out on a lot.[13]

Not everyone can pay or wants to pay for sex. Still, older women are finding other ways to have the intimacy they want without the heteronormative expectations of coupledom and gendered roles. Increasingly, they are embracing friends with benefits relationships (FWB), defined as an ongoing relationship between two people who don't consider themselves a couple that includes sex as well as a level of friendship.[14]

And sometimes those friends are much younger men.

Take Cindy Gallop. Now in her sixties, the ad exec and founder of Make Love, Not Porn only has sex with younger men. Rather than pay for it, the happily and purposefully single woman cultivates relationships with younger men on online sites, she tells me, many of whom she has been with for years. It offers her what she says are ongoing intimate, respectful, and affectionate relationships, and sex when and how she wants it.

Call her a cougar—she owns it, but not in a negative clichéd version of the word.

"I'm very open that I date men casually and recreationally, and I date a lot of them simultaneously. And even I am gobsmacked by the number of younger men who want to meet older women and date older women. They're not all there just to have sex with older women. There are many more younger men who want to date older women than the world thinks. It's just they fear they'll be shamed, or be socially ostracized," if they openly talk about it, she tells me.[15]

What's the attraction, I ask her, knowing in my gut what she tells me to be true.

"I hear this all the time and I really sympathize with this—girls their own age are rampantly insecure, and that's a lot of work, and a lot of emotional wear and tear. They are just enormously drawn to confident women, experienced women, who don't get jealous if they like some woman's Instagram photo."

There is some science backing that up. A 2010 post on the dating app OK Cupid's blog confirms what Gallop is experiencing—older women are more sexual.[16] Not only that, but their data shows that "younger men want to be dominated. Older women are generally interested in doing just that."

"Older women" in this case are women in their thirties and forties—hardly "old" but older than the twenty-somethings many men of any age seem to prefer. But the blog makes it clear: "There are two operative stereotypes of older single women: the sad-sack (à la Bridget Jones) and the 'cougar' (à la Samantha from 'Sex in the City') and both, like all stereotypes, are reductionist and stupid and I've tried to avoid them. I hesitated beginning my case for older women with something about their sexuality . . . because that territory borders right on cougar country. But the evidence there was too compelling to ignore."

Obviously not all younger men want to be intimate with older women or be dominated by them, and not all older women are confident, experienced or "more sexual," but the idea that all women suddenly lose interest in sex as they age, and men lose interest in them, is clearly not what research shows.

DESIRE HAS NO EXPIRATION DATE

In truth, if sex is important to a woman at midlife, she's much more likely to stay sexually active as she ages, even until an age that might surprise—or, sadly, disgust—many.[17] Some 71 percent of hetero women between the ages of eighty and a hundred and two say they still had sexual fantasies or daydreams about men.[18]

Go girls!

Given all that, why do so many still believe that all older women lose interest in sex?

There are a few reasons. There's a general societal belief that older people aren't as interested in sex as much as they used to be, except perhaps men, who we've been told have a higher sex drive than women do. There's also a belief that older people shouldn't care about sex—isn't that just for young people? If a woman buys into that thinking, it's likely she could start to question just how interested in sex she actually is (although it's just as possible that a woman who doesn't have much of an interest in sex might embrace that attitude so she doesn't have to see her ho-hum desire as being a problem).[19]

What researchers have found is that many married women, both hetero and lesbian, just kind of expect that there will be less sex as they age. And they took comfort in that belief—"We're having less sex now because that's just what happens!"[20] Which, of course, grants them a "buy" to not have sex.

Let's be honest, sex can be frustrating or downright painful for menopausal and postmenopausal women. Things happen to a woman's vagina—the vaginal tissue dries out and thins, the vagina itself can narrow and shorten, the pelvic floor muscles start freaking out, and a host of other unpleasantries, all of which can cause so much stress that it may prevent her from enjoying sex. So it's understandable if she starts to avoid it.[21]

A woman could also lose interest in sex if she has health problems; she's depressed; she's on medication that impacts the libido,
like some antidepressants; she's been physically or sexually abused,
or both; or if her romantic relationship isn't so great.[22]
But perhaps the most obvious reason is how society tends to think
about a woman's aging body—she's lost her looks, her body is sagging and wrinkled, she's no longer feminine, she's not desirable,
she's become invisible, it's shameful, it's disgusting, etc.

Even if she feels comfortable in her own aging skin, the messages
are clear. Again, buying into those stereotypes also could lessen a
woman's sexual desire. Having sex "requires an emphasis on the
body, which could become a source of anxiety and depression for
women who are not successful at coping with their bodily changes,"
Maciel and Laganà note.

Anxiety? Depression? It becomes a self-fulfilling prophecy.

Conversely, the researchers say, if a woman has a positive attitude about aging, and sees it as a sign of personal growth and
self-confidence, it could boost her thoughts about her desirability
and even her libido.

Perhaps you can see the problem here. The more society keeps
reinforcing the stereotypes about middle-aged and older women's
sexuality, or more accurately described as our asexuality—what
has distressingly been called "geriatric sexuality breakdown syndrome"[23]—the more likely women at midlife and older will internalize the message and see themselves that way, which may then
interfere with their ability to want or enjoy sex.

It's a vicious cycle.

There are other things that can trip up women's sexuality as they
age. Older Black women who grew up in the 1960s, at the height of
the sexual revolution, Civil Rights Movement, Black Power, and the
legalization of abortion, have had to deal with various offensive and
controlling images—the submissive mammy; the sexually aggressive, male emasculating Black matriarch; the promiscuous Jezebel;
and the sexually loose and immoral welfare queen—that can impact
their sexuality as they age. Often, maintaining the role of being the
matriarch—an important and esteemed familial role that includes
being the family protector—conflicted with their view of themselves
as sexual beings worthy of pleasure.[24]

Older Black women may also have to deal with the internalized messaging of slavery on their sexuality—that once they were

past reproductive age, they were considered useless[25]—as well as a history of rape and abuse, and memories of how negatively they were portrayed during America's shameful segregated past all may interfere with their ability to fully express their sexuality and lessen their desire.[26]

It takes a woman with a strong and healthy image of herself to combat those harmful messages. Thankfully, there are increasingly many more women who feel better about themselves as they age; we're more confident, we know our bodies better, we know what we like sexually and we're not shy about sharing that with our partners. It's all rather sexy, isn't it?

Much of how women operate sexually in this world is not necessarily because we are choosing to live that way, but more because we are constantly being told it's how we women are—that we're "naturally" monogamous, that we prefer intimacy over sex, that we can't handle casual sex, etc. Many women actually like having sex and want to be able to enjoy it for as long as they can. Besides feeling good, study after study indicates that sex can be beneficial to our physical and psychological health.[27]

And many of us are enjoying it as we age. According to the eighth annual "Singles in America" survey in 2018, commissioned by the dating website Match.com, women say they're having their best sex at age sixty-six.[28] I'm not sixty-six yet so I'll have to take their word for it until then. Goals!

Society gets a lot of things wrong about women's lust and desire, as Wednesday Martin details in her 2018 book, *Untrue: Why Nearly Everything We Believe About Women, Lust, and Infidelity Is Wrong and How the New Science Can Set Us Free.* Talking to numerous female sex researchers who are busting those myths, Martin discovers they are uncovering "what science writer Natalie Angier has characterized as 'the multiple layers of compromise and restraint' that sheath female sexuality so thoroughly as to make women strangers to ourselves and our own libidos."[29]

In other words, she concludes, they are helping us to rightfully question everything we've been told, believed, or assumed about what motivates women sexually and what we want from a sexual relationship.

Take those questionable beliefs and assumptions and rub them up against our beliefs about an aging woman's body, and it's understandable if an older woman might fear being naked for the first time with a new partner, or might wonder if her longtime partner is turned off by her wrinkles and age spots, or who would rather not bother with sex because she's internalized the harmful message that older women are not—and worse, *should* not be—sexual beings.

"We interpret the lack of sexual interest as proof that women's sexual drive is inherently less strong," writes Esther Perel in her book *The State of Affairs: Rethinking Infidelity.* "Perhaps it would be more accurate to think that it is a drive that needs to be stoked more intensely and more imaginatively—and first and foremost by her, not only by her partner."[30]

Is it any wonder that a woman might feel limited in her sexual self-expression, which may keep her from talking about or acting on her sexual desires, which could prevent her from getting what she wants, whether finding a new romantic partner or improving whatever romantic partnership she's already in?

This is slowly changing. My generation, the Boomers, pioneered the sexual revolution after the widespread introduction of the birth-control pill and pre-HIV and AIDs days, and we've brought our more sexually liberal beliefs with us as we've aged.[31] Many of us are not done with being sexual beings.

Still, we're going to need more than a sex-positive attitude to maintain our sexual desire into our later years; besides decent health, we need a partner who's interested and interesting (unless we're fine with self-pleasure, which has its own merits), and perhaps an openness to finding different ways to be sexual as our body ages.[32] The last part—being open to "finding different ways to be sexual as our body ages"—matters a lot; if the only sex we are used to is penis-vagina and our partner has erectile issues or we have vaginal pain or lubrication issues, or both, then it could mean the end of sex when all we need is to get creative and explore other erogenous zones.

Not every woman has a good partner, good health, and a good sense of sexual exploration, or even some of that. And some are just not interested in sex even if they do, and there's nothing wrong, bad, or worrisome about that. In fact, there are plenty of older women who say that the overemphasis on sex in Western culture can actually get in the way of those who'd prefer to have less sex or at the very least, other kinds of less-pressure sex than penis-vagina (especially because, as I've already noted, that doesn't always lead a woman to orgasm).[33] Getting older does not necessarily change women's experiences of sensuality and pleasure, just perhaps the way we get them.

That is a world many disabled women know. Some have no or limited use of their genitals, which gives them a much more expansive world of sexual expression.

For Robin Wilson-Beattie, a self-described "queer, femme, fat, disabled, Black, Southern, progressive, and sex-positive" forty-something Gen Xer,[34] sex was not something her doctors discussed with her when she experienced a spinal injury in her early thirties, brought on by a rare birth defect. In fact, many health-care providers assumed she couldn't have sex.[35] So she became a disability and sexuality health educator, writer, and advocate, working toward getting able-bodied people to realize that living with a disability does not take away one's sexual needs and desires.

Differently abled people actually are much more open to finding various ways to be sexual because they sometimes have no other choice.

Beyond hormonal changes, a woman may lose interest in sex at midlife if she hasn't had much pleasure out of it. If a sexually inexperienced woman partnered early—in her teens or early twenties—with one of her first few sexual partners, or perhaps only sexual partner, "it's pretty easy to settle into a pretty subpar erotic life," Chicago psychologist Alexandra H. Solomon tells me. "I have met women who've spent decades faking orgasms, or infrequently having orgasms. That heterosexual sexual script, it just limits women in such profound ways. I can see how it's hard, over time, to keep having subpar sex. And then add in a career, kids, and it's easy to have that become a marginalized part of life."[36]

But sometimes, there's a sexual awakening when a woman least expects it—sometimes after a midlife divorce.

MARITAL DOLDRUMS

Many years ago when I was relatively newly divorced, I was sitting on the sidelines of my younger son's Little League game and a fellow mom sidled up to me and we began to chat. Eventually, it got around to the topic of sex. Do not underestimate how often that subject comes up at youth sports games.

She confided that after X-number of years of marriage, she wasn't really feeling it in the bedroom with her husband, a man I knew and who seemed like a good guy. "I've lost interest in sex," she sighed.

She asked me what it was like to be single at midlife. Since I was in a relationship with a slightly younger man who was rocking my sexual world and postmenopausal zest, I answered honestly. "Great."

She smiled, but I detected a hint of sadness behind it.

What I didn't say and wouldn't say, but most certainly thought, was that if she had a new partner, perhaps a slightly younger man, I'd pretty much bet that she'd get interested in sex ASAP.

And while I didn't know it at the time, research had my back.

According to one study of 438 Australian-born women, the No. 1 thing that boosted a middle-aged woman's libido was having a new sexual partner.[37] That could come in the form of an affair partner, having an open relationship, or consciously uncoupling.

Midlife women who left marriages that were less than sexually satisfying discovered that having new lovers was pretty exciting, even if those relationships were short-lived. Of course, no one is promoting divorce as a path to sexual pleasure. That said, it often is, as researchers Kate A. Morrissey Stahl, Jerry Gale, Denise C. Lewis, and Doug Kleiber found in their small study of hetero, bisexual, and trans divorcees ages fifty-seven to ninety-one. Although a few of the women had some regrets and experienced challenges, divorce got them out of their comfort zone and opened them up sexually.[38]

As the researchers note, "women sometimes have to break rules to find sexual pleasure for themselves in a society which is not consistently supportive of female sexual pleasure. . . . It also takes seriously women's right to seek pleasure and to overcome barriers to pleasure even if those barriers are socially sanctioned."

You shouldn't have to blow up a marriage to get some hot sex. But that doesn't mean that some women don't push the limits anyway.

In her 2018 memoir, *Love and Trouble: A Midlife Reckoning*, Claire Dederer, then fifty-one, confesses to having "extremely inconvenient feelings"—a desire for the recklessness of her youth and a rebooted libido as she hits midlife. "My whole youth was focused on being desired by others and my gosh, it's coming to a close," she told *The Seattle Times*.[39] After some sexless years while raising two children and coming to grips with the fact that she hadn't kissed someone other than her husband in sixteen years, she comes dangerously close to having an affair and blowing up the self-described perfect life she worked so hard to have. Eventually, her husband benefited from her newfound lust.

Ada Calhoun makes out with a man who's not her husband; he's already had an affair by then and shares a kiss with another woman on the night of Calhoun's make-out session, she confesses in her 2017 book, *Wedding Toasts I'll Never Give*. After more than a decade of marriage, a second for both, and at the cusp of midlife, she writes, "When I think about Neal kissing someone else, I want to start knocking things off tables. When I think about myself kissing someone else, I get a thrill."[40]

Author Kim Brooks also starts "acting like the woman I'd been at 21—restless, impulsive and ravenous" in her late thirties. "I yearned and flirted; I had a slew of inappropriate email friendships. I became enamored often and briefly and felt certain these behaviors were a sign there was something wrong with my mental health or my marriage." She wonders if she, too, just wants to be seen by someone other than her husband.[41] Eventually, she and her husband briefly opened up their marriage.[42]

As I was saying, so much for the idea that midlife women lack desire or are undesirable. What is it about women who are ostensibly satisfied with their marriages who want to make out with random men at midlife?

For one, it's expectations. Of marriage.

When my mother married a week shy of her twenty-first birthday in 1950, marriage was just what women did, more out of duty and financial necessity. Women expect a lot more from marriage nowadays, and many struggle with what domesticity and motherhood does to us—what renowned therapist Esther Perel calls the muting of eros in her 2017 book *The State of Affairs: Rethinking Infidelity*, which details the growing number of women seeking sexual satisfaction outside their marriage. Hubby thinks that his wife isn't interested in sex—she keeps rejecting him, after all, or when they finally get around to having sex, she's hoping it's over soon—and so he's stunned when he discovers she's been having a torrid love affair. What the heck is going on?[43]

"Home, marriage and motherhood have forever been the pursuit of many women," Perel writes, "but also the place where women cease to feel like women."[44]

Sound familiar? It does to me. We go from being a desired being to a domestic being and at midlife, we desire to be a desired being again, as Dederer observes.

Being a desired being often becomes a challenge after midlife, not only because women have to fight the narrative that they're no longer desirable, but also because sometimes, stuff happens. It's when many women find themselves becoming caregivers to their typically older spouses or romantic partners, often just at the time that their days of caregiving children, if they have them, may be coming to an end. Not only do they face ageist and sexist beliefs that older women are asexual, but they also find that their new role as a caregiver to their romantic partner becomes all-encompassing. That could hugely impact how a woman feels about her sexuality, even if she had been feeling pretty desirable up until that point.[45]

When we talk about women becoming asexual as they age, it quickly becomes clear that it often happens because of life circumstances—the lack of a sexual partner or an unwilling or unable sexual partner—and not necessarily because it's our choice. And sometimes, it's because, as my Little League mom knows, sex with just one man for many years becomes boring.

What are we to do about that?

ADVENTURES IN NON-MONOGAMY

Maybe you have read the standard evolutionary psychology trope about how men and women have evolved—men need to sow their seed wherever and whenever and to whomever as often as possible, because they can, and women need a partner who's going to hang around long enough to raise her young.

Which means women need to latch onto one man to deliver the goods. Researchers beg to differ, however, arguing that although much of science "may be socially constructed, it is also the case that science is often used as a camouflage for bias in the construction of social life. In other words, that theory contributes to "persistent sexism."[46]

So, the narrative has long been that women not only need a monogamous relationship, but that we prefer it and do better in it. Many researchers—mostly female—are beginning to question that. All you have to do is read the title of their 2014 study to know what Ali Ziegler and associates think about that: "Does Monogamy Harm Women? Deconstructing Monogamy with a Feminist Lens." The researchers, whose work focuses on consensual non-monogamy, explore whether women thrive in monogamy or if alternative relationships, such as polyamory, would better answer the perennial question—what do women want?[47]

What they discovered reveals much. For a large number of women diagnosed with Hypoactive Sexual Desire Disorder, the loss of sexual desire and fantasies is often because she and her partner have mismatched sexual libidos. In other words, it's not just her problem, it's their problem (as with most issues between a couple). They also found that women's desire fades faster than men's in long-term monogamous romantic relationships and that women have a greater need than men for novelty in order to maintain sexual arousal—without it, their sexual desire is likely to diminish. Another finding—polyamory, the practice of having consensual multiple romantic and often sexual relationships, offers women more sexual satisfaction and greater sexual agency.

There's a lot going on in that study. Not every woman at midlife—or at any age, for that matter—may want to become polyamorous, and not every woman loses her desire in her long-term monogamous romantic relationship. Many women actually prefer to have one partner to call their own. That said, some women at midlife feel sexually restless and are more interested in being satisfied in bed and gaining greater sexual agency than new sexual positions, buying sexy lingerie, or planning date nights. And so they are finding workarounds.

Midlife is when women are likely to seek out an affair, not just a one-off make-out session.[48] There are a few reasons why.

Sociologist Alicia M. Walker's research into why women sought flings revealed that for some, it's a way to break free from their limiting and restrictive role as "wife." (It was poet Jill Bialosky who famously said, "I had wanted to get married, but I realized now that I never wanted to be a 'wife.'")[49] For others, it's a way to alleviate whatever fear they have of becoming undesirable. The affairs not only offered them stress relief, Walker discovered, but some also got immense joy in having someone validate and appreciate their body and beauty. And, of course, they had great orgasms.[50]

"Sometimes I wonder if when the kids leave I should either (a) have a passionate affair or (b) find another husband," a friend confesses to author Kim Brooks. "I may do neither, but it seems like (a) is more likely than (b). I don't have any illusions that marrying someone else will make me happy, not anymore."[51]

There are of course other options than illicit trysts with others. For Tessa and Amir (not their real names) it was opening up their marriage of thirty years nearly fourteen years ago, when she was in her late forties and their three children were in high school. "We are the Baby Boomers and Gen Xers who reject the traditional roles that our parents played and the empty nest syndrome. We defy the stigma of ageism, ailing health, empty retirement and a passionless sex life," they write on their website, The Open Nesters.

Opening up their marriage was more of a slow journey than a conscious decision to prepare for their empty-nester stage, but it's brought new sexual energy into this part of their life.

"My expression of myself is very clear about how much I love to be desired and how much that fuels me and how much I want to dress up when someone wants me to. Having someone like that, who wants to see me that way, and . . . wants to court me has really helped Amir to give that to me as well," Tess, a sexuality coach, tells me. "I feel desired and I feel excited and I feel new relationship energy. I can become alive again. It activates my creativity, I feel much juicier, I feel more alive."[52]

And it's a turn-on for Amir to see her that way.

Elle Beau (not her real name), in her mid-fifties, and her husband began seeing other people after twenty-three years of marriage. That was five years ago, when their son was in his teens.

The editor of "Sensual: An Erotic Life," a sex-positive community on the social media platform Medium, she says her sexual awakening didn't really kick in until she was fifty. "Getting older gave us both the confidence and the desire to explore and expand our horizons."[53]

Even before they opened up their marriage, they had hit a sweet spot because they had each come into their own bodies. This comes with age, she writes. "Middle-aged and older women tend to have a better sense of who they really are perhaps because they've finally given up at least some of trying to be who the world told them they should be. That means they are more self-confident, both inside and outside of the bedroom. Self-confident women are both more relaxed and more willing to try new things."[54]

Trying new things could take many forms, some that may even be surprising.

SOMETHING DIFFERENT

"Dear Ones. There is something I wish to tell you today—something which I hope and trust you will receive with grace," began Elizabeth Gilbert's *Facebook* post on Sept. 7, 2016. In describing the terminal cancer diagnosis of her dear friend of sixteen years, Rayya Elias, Gilbert made a confession: "I do not merely love Rayya; I am in love with Rayya."

It was another surprise in the evolution of the author of *Eat, Pray, Love,* the best-selling 2006 book and then movie that became like a bible for middle-aged women who left husbands and jobs to find their passion and adventure. The announcement came just months after another bombshell confession—that she was separating from her husband, José Nunes, aka "Felipe," the love part of her memoir.[55]

Gilbert is hardly the first heterosexual woman to become attracted to women later in life. Around the same time that Gilbert was professing her love for Elias, Glennon Doyle, author of the best-selling book *Love Warrior* among others and creator of the popular online community Momastery, famously left her husband of fourteen years and, a year later, married soccer icon and Olympian Abby Wambach.

Those are just two recent high-profile examples, but research shows that some 36 percent of women in their forties in a same-sex relationship had been previously married to men. It's higher for women in their fifties and older.[56]

There wasn't much research on the phenomenon until Nancy C. Larson's 2006 article "Becoming 'One of the Girls,'" in which she discovered that coming out at midlife—something she herself did after nineteen years of marriage to a man—was a huge boost to women's libido. "[M]any women report feeling a "second adolescence," with many of the associated feelings and behaviors. She is not crazy if she suddenly has sex on the brain all the time!"[57]

Since then, more, mostly female, researchers have been exploring late-life same-sex attraction, most notably University of Utah professor Lisa M. Diamond. Diamond has been following 100 women who report some same-sex attraction but who sometimes change the way they describe themselves—gay, straight, or bisexual—which Diamond calls "sexual fluidity." Often, that fluidity appears later in life.

"What we know about adult development suggests that people become more expansive in a number of ways as they get older," Diamond told *The Guardian* in 2010, after her book, *Sexual Fluidity: Understanding Women's Love and Desire,* was published. "I think a lot of women, late in life, when they're no longer worried about raising the kids, and when they're looking back on their marriage and how satisfying it is, find an opportunity to take a second look at what they want and feel like."[58]

That, she says, may be frightening for some but exciting and quite liberating for others. "[T]he notion that your sexuality can undergo these really exciting, expansive possibilities at a stage when most people assume that women are no longer sexually interesting and are just shutting down, is potentially a really liberating notion for women. Your sexual future might actually be pretty dynamic and exciting—and whatever went on in your past might not be the best predictor at all of what your future has in store."

Perhaps, as the North American Menopause Society suggests, having a male sexual partner isn't really all that necessary once a woman's postmenopausal.[59]

Sorry, guys!

As for lesbian "bed death," Paige Averett, a North Carolina State University professor who researches LGBTQ and minorities issues, finds that some older lesbians tend to place more value on the emotional aspects of a romantic relationship than on sex. They're not getting it on any more or less than hetero women are, but again, having a positive attitude about getting older was linked to enjoying sex more and having more of it.[60]

So, what if you're not all that interested in sex for whatever reason, or unable to have the kind of sex you'd like for whatever reason. Perhaps all of the above has you questioning if there's something wrong with you. There isn't, of course. Yet the discourse of the "new aging" movement, with its emphasis on aging success-fully (more on that in chapter 6) is within everyone's ability and desire no matter their circumstances could certainly make someone feel that way.[61] Feeling like you have to be sexually active well into old age may put unnecessary pressure on women to do whatever it takes to maintain a functional body and healthy libido so they can be a "sexy ageless consumer," which would require us to purchase products, prescriptions, or procedures.[62]

That sounds exhausting and expensive, a discussion we'll explore in more depth in chapter 4.

DON'T ASK, DON'T TELL

After she experienced marriage to a man who had no interest in sex, Dr. Jen Gunter began listening differently to the women she cared for in her OB-GYN practice in San Francisco.

"There are spaces between words that tell entire stories. When I ask someone about her sex life and there is a pause or a generic 'O.K.,' I say, 'You know, the libido issue is often with the man,'" she writes in her health column in the *New York Times*. "The responses from women are so similar that I could script it. A pause, then relief that it's not just them, followed quickly by the desire to hear more. Many tell me intimate details, so glad to have someone in whom they can confide."[63]

If you have a doctor as conscientious as Dr. Gunter, you are lucky. Many doctors struggle with bringing up the topic of sex with their older patients. Sometimes it's because they just lack knowledge about later-in-life sex, but they also often assume that sex is less important to older women and maybe not important at all. So, they often prefer that their patients bring up the subject first. This creates a problem for some older women who fear talking openly with their health-care provider because they feel like they'll be judged for being sexually active, or at least having an interest in it, "at their age."[64] There's a lot of stigma around later-life sex, which leaves many older women's concerns underreported, ignored, or left untreated.

This is especially true for older Mexican-American women, who make up a substantial portion of the older Hispanics in the United States. Talking about sexual concerns or unmet sexual needs with a health-care provider could possibly lead to vergüenza (sexual shame) or culpa (guilt), especially in a culture where a woman's sexuality in later years or outside of a church-sanctified marriage is frowned upon.[65]

As a disabled woman, Wilson-Beattie says hitting midlife has proved challenging.

"What no one talks about is aging with a chronic condition, and how it affects you physically, and mentally. Perimenopause is currently here, signaling the end of my reproductive cycle. The change of hormones means my libido and sexual needs have started to change," she writes in an essay on *Pulp*.[66]

Libido and sexual needs change throughout a woman's life. That's the narrative we need to embrace. Dr. Holly N. Thomas, an assistant professor of medicine at the University of Pittsburgh, focuses her research on the various factors that can create sexual issues for women at midlife and beyond. After following 3,200 women for nearly fifteen years, Thomas and her team discovered that the myth that women lose their sexual appetite at midlife is just that—a myth.

Although nearly half said they slowly began to lose interest at midlife (see above for the possible reasons why), 27 percent said an active sex life was very important to them throughout their forties, fifties, and sixties. Midlife sex is not abnormal, Thomas notes.[67]

No, it's not. But Thomas goes on to say something that to me seems to be key: "If women are able to speak up with their partner and make sure that they're having sex that's fulfilling and pleasurable to them, then they're more likely to rate it as highly important as they get older."

The problem is, women don't always speak up. Of course, we also live in a culture that does not place much—if any—emphasis on women's sexual pleasure, as I note above, and not only doesn't encourage it, but often diminishes, dismisses, and ignores it all while perpetuating myths about women's sexuality as we age.

So where does that leave us? We could wait until someone comes along who knows what they're doing to have the kind of pleasure we deserve, as Eve's mom unexpectedly experienced at age ninety-one. Or we can speak up and change that narrative right now.

THINGS TO THINK ABOUT

How important is sex to you?
How have you experienced sex and pleasure as you've aged?
In what ways do you believe people get "too old" for sex?
What would you want to change about your sex life?
What kind of sex life would you want to have at midlife and beyond?

3

I Do, I Don't, I Won't

[W]hy has modern love developed in such a way as to maximize submission and minimize freedom, with so little argument about it?

— Laura Kipnis, *Against Love*

Emma Watson created a stir when, shortly before her thirtieth birthday in 2019, she declared herself "self-partnered." It wasn't something she was necessarily embracing. In fact, she didn't believe women actually could be happy all by themselves. No, she was pretty sure women needed a romantic partner and had to have one by a certain age—thirty—and get on with things.

"I was like, 'Why does everyone make such a big fuss about turning 30? This is not a big deal. . . . Cut to 29, and I'm like, 'Oh my God, I feel so stressed and anxious. And I realise it's because there is suddenly this bloody influx of subliminal messaging around," she said in an interview in the U.K. *Vogue,* "If you have not built a home, if you do not have a husband, if you do not have a baby, and you are turning 30, and you're not in some incredibly secure, stable place in your career, or you're still figuring things out. . . . There's just this incredible amount of anxiety."[1]

I feel for Emma and her peers.

Let's imagine Emma's self-partnering doesn't last all that long. Say she's now in her forties or fifties, married and mom to a child or

49

two, maybe stepmom to a child or two as well. She has everything she thinks she wants, or what society tells her she *should* want—will she be content or will she find herself questioning her life as authors Claire Dederer and Ada Calhoun did, or questioning monogamy as Tessa and Elle Beau did, or discover her sexual fluidity like Elizabeth Gilbert and Glennon Doyle have, all of which we explored in chapter 2? Will she find herself among the growing numbers of couples consciously uncoupling in their fifties or later, once the kids are grown and their "job" as parents is basically done? Will she stay married, happily or unhappily? Or will she find herself suddenly widowed, and once again, self-partnered and maybe this time fully embracing it after years of "been there, done that" as a wife?

There's no way to know, of course. But in a world filled with Disney fairy-tale romance and Hollywood rom-coms, it's hard to escape the pull of romantic love, commitment, and marriage, especially for hetero women. It's what philosopher Elizabeth Brake calls "amatonormativity"—the belief that everyone desires an exclusive, romantic, long-term coupled relationship, and the pressure that puts on women to be partnered and stay partnered.[2]

Even as society pushes romantic partnering, especially in the form of marriage, on girls and women in their twenties and thirties, it sends a different message to single, divorced, and widowed women at midlife and beyond: Sorry! You're too old to find love again, no one even sees you (damn that invisibility!), and anyway, why would anyone want you when they can have a younger, prettier, possibly more sexual version?

We've come a long way from the *Newsweek* cover in June 1986 that proclaimed that if a woman hadn't tied the knot by age forty, well, good luck—she'd be more likely to be killed by a terrorist. The article, "Too Late for Prince Charming," and the research on which it had been based, have long since been debunked, causing the news magazine to retract it twenty years later. Still, it had entrenched itself in our collective consciousness. As journalist Megan Garber writes in *The Atlantic* in 2016, "what's perhaps most striking about the story, 30 years later, is how oddly fresh it still feels, how urgent its anxieties still seem. The piece's core message—panic, ladies, because your professional goals will undermine your personal ones—lives on, in its way, in every current news story about the difficulty educated women face in the 'marriage market,' in every blithe reference to the 'biological clock,' and indeed in every piece of media that gazes upon women's bodies and sees, in their fleshy fallibility, some form of social determinism."[3]

Amatonormativity is also what makes women who are single, whether by choice or chance, feel marginalized and become, in the eyes of many, crazy cat ladies—a trope that must have nine lives because it refuses to die.

Yet women are more likely than men to be single for a greater portion of their lives, even the hetero women who follow the romantic script, marry, and have children. The vast majority of hetero women marry men who are older than they are, which leaves many of them widows at a relatively young age—the average age of widowhood in America is a mere fifty-nine years old, according to the Census Bureau.[4] That leaves decades of living ahead.

Whatever will happen to them?

Hopefully, whatever they want.

For one, many of those widows have no desire to marry again, and not always because they believe no man can take their former husband's place (although some feel strongly about that). Some are no longer interested in the highly gendered package deal that often comes with marriage—all the homemaking and caregiving, and having to schedule much of their lives around a new hubby and his interests.[5] Some say they don't want to grieve over losing yet another spouse while others do not want to give up their newfound freedom, both of which sound totally understandable. And some, as Regina Kenen, a widowed sociologist, discovered, flat-out admit they don't "find older men, in general, to be very interesting or attractive. They found women to be better companions."[6]

Sorry guys!

Another damaging reality of amatonormativity is that it often leads women (and men, too) to seemingly the worst fate that could ever possibly befall them—dying alone. And the fear of dying alone has kept many women in unhealthy or unsatisfying romantic relationships.[7]

It's an irrational fear, of course, as so many fears are. Still, it's OK to be fearful, as long as fear doesn't drive your choices. Sadly, it often does. And while it may appear to be more likely that the married and/or living together couples among us *may* have a loved one nearby at the moment when death arrives, there's no guarantee that they *will* be there. It's just as likely that a non-romantic partner, friend, roomie, co-worker, parent, or child will be close by at the moment we need them most—or nobody.

Just look at the late Supreme Court Justice Antonin Scalia. Despite having a wife of fifty-six years, nine children and thirty-six grand-children, Scalia died doing what he loved, hunting, but alone. Whatever fear he may or may not have had about going this way, instead of being surrounded by his loved ones in his own bed, he died far from home; even the members of the secretive male-only hunting group he was with at a west Texas ranch weren't nearby.[8]

What is it about dying alone that causes so much fear when we actually should fear settling for decades in an unsatisfying life, which is a heck of a lot longer than the moments right before death? In part, that's the narrative. People who die alone are seen as having "bad deaths," even if that may be someone's preferred way of going. For whatever reason, we equate dying alone with loneli-ness although being alone is not the same as being lonely.[9] As we've learned during the coronavirus pandemic, many of those who died from COVID-19 weren't able to have loved ones by their side—did all those people live lonely lives? Of course not.

So, the narrative is wrong. It's time to say, "Rest in peace" to it.

In truth, many partnered women will find themselves alone at midlife and beyond, either through divorce or widowhood. That's a reality all women need to think about. How will we handle it? What will we do differently?

There are numerous stereotypes about women and love at this stage of our life that are damaging—not only for single women, whether never married, divorced, or widowed women, but also for married women. Most of them promote the belief that women are much more relationship oriented than men are; therefore, all women "need" or "want" a romantic partner. Some judge women who leave their romantic partners (often quite harshly). Others are warned to keep themselves looking young and fit so their husbands don't ditch them for a younger woman or cheat on them. (Note: you cannot "affair-proof" a marriage, no matter what the so-called relationship experts say, because you can't, and shouldn't have to, control your partner's behavior.) A lot of those stereotypes and judgments have to do with the societal pressure women feel to be in that "exclusive, romantic, long-term coupled relationship," and do whatever they can to maintain it, even if it comes at great cost to them.

At the same time, older women who may want a romantic partner and sex (please revisit chapter 2 if you need a refresher) are told, nah, not happening for you, Granny. You're too old.

It often seems like we gals just can't win.

What if women weren't so driven by the fear of dying, or aging, alone? What if being self-partnered was nothing to fear, but something to actually celebrate? What if we recognized that finding new romantic partners and even marriage, if we want that, has no age limit? What if we didn't have to feel that we are "less than" because we're single? What if we didn't fear the shame and judgment of feeling unsatisfied in a romantic relationship? What if we asked ourselves, "What kind of love and companionship do I want—if any—as I age?" What would we do differently in our life? What kind of relationships would we nurture; what kind of relationships would we free ourselves from?

Let's talk about it.

IS THAT ALL THERE IS?

Honestly, being single at midlife was not what I expected. I did marry twice, after all—a starter marriage when I was way too young, not even twenty-one, and again at age thirty-two, each time with the expectation of happily ever after. One of those marriages should have lasted, right? What about "until death do we part" did I not understand? Clearly, something must be wrong with me because I can't "keep" a man—never mind that I, or any other woman for that matter, just may not want to have a poorly matched partner hang around.

Although I didn't dream of being swept away by a prince to live happily ever after in a castle somewhere as a young girl, I did grow up with some romantic notions and a society-approved script of what my life "should" look like—meet, date, fall in love, marry, house, a couple of kids. No one warned me there might be a minivan as well. (I ditched it a few years after my divorce.)

And I did have that in my second marriage, except for the "ever after" part. When I found myself single at midlife, that old romantic script didn't work anymore. I didn't "need" a husband for kids or a house or financial stability—I already had all that. Did I "need" a husband? (No.) Did I even "need" a man at all? (Well, as a hetero cis woman I wasn't ready to give up sex quite yet so, no, I didn't *need* one, but, yes, I *wanted* one.) But it took me four decades to ask myself for the first time in my life, "Vicki, what do you want?" Once I actually sat down with myself to think about it, some things became clearer, others remain muddled and open to interpretation.

There is no script, society approved or not, for women middle-aged and older. This is both challenging and liberating. We have to create it ourselves. Or toss the idea of a script away entirely and make it up as we go along. I prefer to be more intentional at this point in my life; I don't want to waste a lot of time.

Still, that does not stop people from perpetuating relationship myths about women like me and, I am guessing since you picked up this book, most likely you.

When I look at women around my age, midlife and older, I see that they, too, are asking themselves, what do I want? They are craving something more.

Some are single by choice or chance, others are married but there is often something that is making them feel restless, too. It isn't quite the "problem that has no name" that Betty Friedan spoke about decades ago in her seminal book *The Feminine Mystique.* Today's women, with all the options available to us, are beyond that. But as we hit midlife and older, with a heightened sense of mortality, when science says women's happiness disappears[10] (it comes back, trust me), we often find ourselves asking, "Is this all there is?"

The answer is no.

If we block the noise of what our life "should" look like at this age and instead focus on what we would like it to look like, now and moving forward, we open ourselves to the many possibilities that exist, or that we can create. Remember, we are talking about our future self, and we want to be as kind and loving to her as we often feel when we look back at our teenaged self and wish we could give her a hug while tenderly telling her, "Oh, lovely, you're going to be OK."

Not to say that's easy. While we've seen a huge expansion of how women have been shaping their lives in recent years, many of us still carry an internal dialogue that says we can't or shouldn't do X, Y, or Z and only can or should do X, Y, or Z. And even if we can fight that dialogue within us, there are many others—even some of our closest friends and family—who will judge us if we move too far from their comfort level. At some point, though, there is a desire, maybe even a sense of urgency, to live a life that's more true to ourselves.

That's what Vanessa D. Fabbre, an assistant professor at the George Warren Brown School of Social Work, discovered in her study of trans men who transitioned to women in their fifties and later. They followed society's dictates, did all the things they were "supposed" to do, and then realized that there's only so much time left to live. "An acute perception that there are limited days in which to embrace one's authentic self, experience the joy of feeling whole and congruent within oneself and to face death with a sense of having truly lived is central to the contemplation of transition for many people," she writes.[11]

Not surprisingly, coming out later in life creates a kind of "second adolescence" for trans women—they're exploring dating, sex, and romantic relationships for the first time as a woman if they're single, although sometimes their explorations are within a heterosexual marriage.[12]

If you've been married for any length of time and are at the "Is this all there is?" phase, you may see only two options—divorce or stay and continue with more of the (often miserable) same.

Marital distress at midlife is real, says San Francisco Bay Area psychologist Daphne de Marneffe, who calls this marital period "the rough patch" in her 2018 book by the same name. A lot of de Marneffe's book addresses the individual development that she sees as essential to get through this seemingly inevitable period in a long-term partnership.

Still, that often isn't enough, she tells me. Sometimes, as hard as it may seem, divorce really is the best decision.

"I had this idea that if people really took themselves on and looked into themselves and worked on themselves and healed themselves, that that would be the critical thing to make for a happy marriage. And I do believe that," she says. "But I also believe that sometimes when you do all that, where you end up is realizing, 'This marriage can't work' or, 'I feel this marriage is too limited.' I had this kind of simplistic view that if you do all that work, you would be able to work it out. And of course that's ridiculous because there are two people."[13]

Right, there are two people and both have to be equally invested to keep a marriage going. Just as you can't affair-proof a marriage, you can't divorce-proof one either because you can't control another person's behavior; you can only control your own. All you can do is be the best person you can be in your marriage because you want to be the best person, period, and hope your spouse does the same.[14]

That may explain why we are seeing such a rise in divorce among people ages fifty and older, which doubled between 1990 and 2010.[15] And it's even grown since then.[16] The stereotype has generally been that men ditch their wives at midlife for a younger woman.[17] And while that does indeed occur at times, in truth, women are much more likely to seek divorce than men are.[18]

Jocelyn Elise Crowley, a professor of public policy at Rutgers University, thought the overwhelming reason for the high rate of divorce among Boomers—the generation that grew up in the by-now clichéd self-empowered, self-actualizing, make-love-not-war 1960s—would be because they were no longer feeling fulfilled in their marriage. This is often the narrative of conservatives who believe that couples split too easily and for the "wrong" reasons (and, I ask, based on whose definition of "wrong"?), and why there has been a movement to make divorce harder in the United States, even though research shows making divorce easier and cheaper is better for everyone, especially women. How much better? There are far fewer cases of women dying by suicides or experiencing domestic violence, and that alone is enough.[19] What she discovered was something entirely different—Boomers divorced for "surprisingly old-fashioned reasons." True, some indicated they'd just grown apart, or there was infidelity (that happens a lot because, let's face it, monogamy can be hard for some people) or mental health issues.

But, she learned, women were unhappy with their husbands' addictions, whether to alcohol, drugs, or pornography, or some combination thereof. Many said their husbands were emotionally or verbally abusive, often for years, and at some point, they decided they'd had enough.[20]

So, it's not like Boomers simply want "to spread their wings because they are no longer fulfilled, or 'hippies gone wild.' Instead, this mid-life population takes splitting up very seriously and, more often than not, considers whether their promised binding responsibilities to each other have been violated when they file for divorce," she writes.

Exactly. Because it's a secret that actually isn't a secret: Women generally don't up and leave satisfying, healthy, and loving relationships. Why would we?

But for those couples who actually feel like they've grown apart, or who are veering close to the edge—and the coronavirus pandemic has exacerbated the number of couples at that point[21]—there may indeed be possibilities.

We already saw in chapter 2 how some couples have been able to reconnect at midlife and revive their sex life by opening up their marriage—a decision, again, often driven by the women. That may not be an attractive option for you. Admittedly, that's probably a hard one for many people, me included. That's fine. Thankfully, it's not the only way to reconnect. Sometimes, a longtime marriage just needs a reboot.

A reboot is different than going to marital counseling, not that there's anything wrong with that, or taking romantic getaways, having date nights, or buying sexy lingerie to revive a midlife marriage. It's about asking yourself, *what do I want now, with decades of postmenopausal zest ahead of me? Can I get my (perhaps long-ignored or diminished) needs met without having to blow up my marriage?*

Some bold women are making it happen.

I LOVE YOU, NOW GO HOME

As a Boomer, my midlife experience was much different than my mother's. I had so many more choices available to me than she did, when marriage was a woman's ticket—often the only one—to the so-called good life, making us financially dependent on men, and all the damage that arrangement has caused women (more on that in chapter 7).

When I was about to divorce for the second time, I had a heart-to-heart talk with her about marriage and motherhood. Did she like being a mother and wife? Was there anything she regretted?

"Yes," she said in her Romanian accent, still thick despite having left her native country decades earlier, a concentration camp survivor who'd been orphaned at age sixteen in the Holocaust. "I wish I had an affair on your father."

OK, that was *not* what I had expected to hear.

My mother was in her early seventies then and still a stunning woman. For all I knew, my father, whom she married a week before her twenty-first birthday, was the only man she'd had sex with. I knew that my mother was not the only woman my father had sex with, including at least two affairs during their sixty-one-year marriage, although she did not discover them until her sixties.

My mom and I bonded over cooking, sewing, crafts, and (unintentionally) infidelity.

I am sure she had opportunities to stray—with a sly smile she admitted to having "a chance"—especially since she had basically been living on her own. She left our New York City home, bought a condo in Miami, where my sister was living, got herself a job, and created a life for herself independent of my father. They lived apart for about ten years, although my father visited for a long weekend each month, until he retired and permanently joined her in Florida.

I'm pretty sure that's why their marriage lasted that long. Still, it wasn't what my friends' mothers were doing. In fact, I didn't know any woman who willingly lived apart from her spouse.

"What was that all about?" I asked her during that heart-to-heart talk. She had split for Miami when I was in my early twenties, newly married to my first husband, living in Colorado, and not really paying too much attention to what my parents were doing.

"I'd had enough," was all she said. As a mother and former wife of many years myself by that point, I knew *exactly* what she meant. Men hate to hear this, but heterosexual marriage has overwhelmingly been a much better deal for men than it has been for women.[22] As sociologist Lisa Wade notes and study after study confirms, "Women on average do more of the unpaid and undervalued work of households, they work more each day, and they are more aware of this inequality than their husbands. They are more likely to sacrifice their individual leisure and career goals for marriage. Marriage is a moment of subordination and women, more so than men, subordinate themselves and their careers to their relationship, their children, and the careers of their husbands."[23]

Sound familiar?

Thankfully, women are demanding more from marriage now—if they even still want to wed, that is. Yes, they often want the financial perks marriage offers, but many also want emotional support from their spouse, and more equitable sharing of household chores, childcare, and all the other labor women typically do but that all too often goes unnoticed or unappreciated. In other words, they want a true partner, not one in name only.[24] Same-sex couples seem to be able to do this much better than hetero couples, in part because there are fewer gendered expectations.[25]

My mother's generation did not always have that option, and they certainly didn't grow up expecting that they would, so who could blame my mom for wanting something else?

My mother was in her late forties at the time and with her daughters grown, she was truly in her prime, her postmenopausal zest. And she was willing to shake up her comfortable life to take care of herself.

Although she didn't have an affair, she did something as exciting, perhaps even more so, for a woman of her generation—a 1950s stay-at-home suburban mom. At midlife, she created a room of her own, a rich, satisfying life filled with friends, her career, her hobbies, her daughters, and, most important, a new sense of freedom. And, presumably, she enjoyed a lusty long weekend with my father on his monthly visits.

What my mom did was transform her marriage into a live apart together (LAT) arrangement, certainly not a new phenomenon but a growing one in recent years, especially among midlife and older couples.

Can you guess who is driving it? Yep, it's overwhelmingly women, many of whom want that proverbial room of their own.

LAT relationships have been called the "gender revolution continuing into old age," a nod to the fact that Boomer women have been on the forefront of the restructuring of family life in the past few decades.[26]

While many older, heterosexual men prefer to live with their romantic partner, many older women treasure their newfound independence as widows or divorcees or empty nesters after having done the bulk of the housekeeping and caregiving and, if they have children, child-rearing, as women typically do. As my mom did. As I do.

"They've had careers, they're liberated and they're not dependent on the guy," says David Cravit, author of *The New Old: How the Boomers Are Changing Everything . . . Again*. "When they hit this age, they're not going to revert back to being their mothers and their grandmothers."[27]

Diane Burke is one of them. In her late sixties, Burke lives apart from her husband of forty-plus years most of the year; he's in Massachusetts, she's in North Carolina. It was a gradual process, starting in her fifties, she tells me, when she began to have strong yearnings for being in nature, solitude, and freedom—not from her marriage per se, but from her roles and responsibilities as wife and mom to three. She began taking solo trips and when her last child graduated from high school in 2006, Burke bought a small condo in the mountains. Since then, she has spent more time in North Carolina than in New England, which she admits hasn't always made her husband happy.

Although he retired in 2019 at age seventy, there are no plans for him to move to North Carolina. If he did, she says, they'd probably continue to live apart.

"We have had a caring and mutually supportive relationship," she writes in an email. "Because of our long history together, our foundation, and some overlapping values, we have been mostly open and supportive of each other's choices and decisions over the years. (E)ven through the bumps . . . we are interested in staying in a form of a relationship with each other. We continue to be practically and emotionally connected and caring and supportive in ways that add to each other's lives."[28]

Of course, couples don't have to be married to live apart. In fact, many older widows, divorcees, and never-married women with romantic partners are gravitating to this way of living, leading some sociologists and gerontologists to consider it an ideal lifestyle for older men and women.

My friend Sharon Hyman, a Montreal filmmaker in her fifties who's making a documentary on LATs, whom she calls apartners, and who runs a lively and growing *Facebook* page by the same name of which I am a member, knows why. Her relationship with her apartner of more than twenty years offers them the best of both worlds—all the reasons people seek a romantic partner, such as love, commitment, sex, and caregiving, without the 24/7 togetherness and gendered realities of living under one roof.

"I want to live a single life with you. For our couple life would be the equivalent of our single lives today, but together," Canadian writer Isabelle Tessier wrote in a *HuffPost* article, "I Want To Be Single But With You," that went viral. In it, she expressed a desire to have all the joys of a committed relationship but without giving up her freedom and sense of self that being in a relationship often takes away, or at least diminishes.[29]

This has been my preferred way of being in a relationship for the past fifteen years—although I came to that decision slowly—for exactly the desire Tessier expresses.

As Cornell Law School professor Cynthia Grant Bowman notes, LAT relationships are a pretty attractive lifestyle for older people because it allows them "to keep their own familiar space, preserve their inheritance for their children, and, in the case of women, protect themselves against gendered divisions of domestic labor characteristic of marriage."[30]

Let me step it back. I can hear married women, especially Gen X women, asking, how? How can women in their forties right now, in this pandemic-fueled economically disastrous moment after having graduated into the Great Recession, and then dealing with everything that followed, possibly do what my mother did when she hit midlife—set up an entire household separate from the one they might be struggling to hang onto? I hear you. It's an important question, one I would ask myself. And that I actually do ask myself, because honestly, my life would be so much easier (aka cheaper) if I were sharing the ever-increasing costs of living with someone else, whether a romantic partner or a roommate.

With that in mind, there's only one way to answer that question, and (perhaps sadly), it's with a question—what are you willing to do to make your marriage better suit you and your needs right now, to give each other the space you may be craving? The stresses of living and working from home together 24/7 during the pandemic, if that has been your experience, has led some to think a bump in divorces is inevitable once things get back to some sort of sense of normal.[31] Because here's an important thing to acknowledge if you're feeling stifled in your relationship—very few couples remain in the same housing situation once they divorce, meaning each of you will have to find a way to live separately. Why wouldn't that be a consideration if it offered a way to keep your partnership intact?

NO PARTNER, NO KIDS, JUST CATS?

But not every woman is married, widowed, or divorced in her forties, fifties, or sixties and older nowadays. Many are single and increasingly single by choice, not chance. But regardless of whether a woman prefers to fly solo or not, there's a phrase to describe her—a crazy cat lady.

Poor Susan Boyle stepped into that fray when, in 2009, the forty-seven-year-old Scottish singer appeared on the popular television show *Britain's Got Talent*. The audiences and judges sniggered at the somewhat dowdy-looking middle-aged Boyle, who confessed she had never been kissed. But when she sang the first notes of "I

Dreamed a Dream" from "Les Misérables," the sniggering stopped, jaws dropped, and audience and judges alike rose to their feet in enthusiastic applause.

Despite that enthusiastic reaction, the media was merciless, describing her as a "singing spinster" who "lives alone in a row house with her cat Pebbles, a drab existence in one of Scotland's poorest regions. She cared for her widowed mother for years, never married and sang in church and at karaoke nights at the pub."[32]

An unmarried woman with a cat who lives a "drab existence" (according to whom we don't know, but it certainly wasn't how Boyle described her life) can only mean one thing—she's a cat lady, a term that often describes an older asexual woman who lives alone, but she could just as easily be a career woman who "can't seem to find a man," or perhaps isn't interested in one.

Boyle has done quite well without one (although she had a short-lived romance at age fifty-three)—she's a multimillionaire with a thriving singing career, a cameo role in a movie, a musical about her life, an autobiography, a proposed biopic, and an inspiring role model for autistic people everywhere.[33]

If that's being a "cat lady," I have no problem with that.

While "cat lady" may be a negative thing for a hetero woman, the label has been embraced by many lesbians[34] as well as at least one drag queen.[35] "The independence of cats is one of the main parallels between cats and lesbians—women who simply in being lesbians declare themselves untamed in at least some small way," Shoney Sien writes in the introduction to the 1991 anthology *Cats (and Their Dykes).*[36]

Adds oral historian Irene Reti, the book's editor, "There is something between cats and women that is not based on domination or condescending adoration. Cat is telling us about independent grace, beauty born of self-respect and pride. Cat knows how to say when she doesn't want to be touched. Cat knows how to ignore men."

Perhaps knowing how to "ignore men" is a cat lady's superpower. Add that to our "invisibility cloak" and now we're getting somewhere.

WELCOME TO THE F*CK IT YEARS

In Sweden, the idea of "tant," a Swedish word derived from the French word for "aunt," tante, is gaining favor. While it's not quite the same as being a cat lady, it has similar negative connotations—it's used to describe a hefty, matronly, invisible, sexless, and frumpish older woman—but it can also refer to a woman who dares to speak her mind without giving a thought to pleasing others.[37]

And if that doesn't capture exactly what this phase of life for women is about, I don't know what does. At this point, many of us would like to start pleasing ourselves, thank you very much.

In her study of Swedish women aged forty-five to sixty-five, researcher Karin Lövgren discovered that most of the women said their self-esteem increased with age. "One becomes more confident, more aware of one's own opinions, and more secure in standing up for and expressing these—qualities that have traditionally been ascribed to the tant."

And because of that, young Swedish women are celebrating the concept, admiring the idea of being a woman who speaks her truth, and welcoming the idea of being free from the male gaze—what one might call "the f*ck it years."

Isn't there a bit of tant and cat lady in all of us?

Katie Sullivan Barak notes in her doctorate dissertation that "cat lady" is among the many terms throughout history that seek to reinforce dominant gender narratives—women need to adhere to heteronormative gender expectations or else. "[R]epresentations of the crazy cat lady, the reprehensible animal hoarder, the proud spinster, and the unproductive old maid negatively frame independent, single women as models of failed White womanhood," she writes.[38]

With beginnings in witchcraft, the term has been transformed into a stereotype that refuses to die—that lonely, unwanted, embittered single women prefer cats to romantic partners and are thus worthy of pity and ridicule and maybe even disgust.

But calling a woman a cat lady appears to be less about a woman actually *owning* cats, and more about shaming and judging any woman who challenges traditional gendered roles and prefers her independence.

How dare she! Doesn't she know her place?

Clearly women, especially single women, are scrutinized and judged. Once again, research comes to our rescue. A recent study on cat ladies finds that there's no evidence supporting the stereotype: "cat-owners did not differ from others on self-reported symptoms of depression, anxiety or their experiences in close relationships."[39]

To which I say, meow.

I'm pretty sure that women who live with cats already knew that, but thanks anyway. It's unlikely to stop people—well, men—from shaming and judging women who have no interest in fitting into society's view of what we "should" do.

In the meantime, the persistent caricature can prevent many single women from developing a healthy self-image and undermine their self-respect and how they perceive their contribution to society, while also largely ignoring the fact that they are part of a growing and powerful solo sisterhood.[40]

Isn't it time for women to decide what we want to do and not have to doubt those choices, no judgy "shoulds" necessary?

Here's why—about a third of Boomers are single, the vast majority because they're divorced or they never married; just 10 percent are widowed.[41] For Gen Xers, 55 percent have never been married and 33 percent are divorced.[42] And many of them have no children, either by choice or chance.

As much as single women are suspect, so, too, are childfree and childless women, maybe even more so. After all, aren't women "naturally" maternal? Actually, no.

Nearly a quarter of Americans age sixty-five or over don't have a spouse or partner or children to look after them, giving rise in recent years to a horrific title—"elder orphans."[43] But it's not just Boomers. Some 43 percent of Gen X women don't have children.[44] We can expect that number to grow, as fewer women than ever are having babies.[45]

The rise in childfree women seems to bother just about everyone but the women themselves (except, obviously, the women who wanted to have children but didn't or couldn't), who are often warned that they'll regret it later in life (ignoring the reality that some women wanted children, but didn't or couldn't have them for a variety of reasons), they won't be as happy or have the same sense of life purpose as moms have, or they'll be lonely and depressed. Research does not bear out any of that.[46] Nevertheless, women aging without children or partners are exhausted by having to constantly explain why, resulting in an "unsettling blend of being unseen and yet on occasion, being closely scrutinised and subjected to impertinent and intrusive questioning."[47]

Keturah Kendrick is one of those single, childfree women. The Gen Xer has known she didn't want a husband or children since she was young. The author of *No Thanks: Black, Female, and Living in the*

Martyr-Free Zone, Kendrick has heard the "S" word—selfish—a lot because of her choices. She's among the 40 percent of single Black women who are looking for love—on her own terms, she says—but aren't actively dating.[48]

"What's become increasingly more important to me in my 40s are my autonomy and my ability to be free. The best thing about being single is being able to shape my life the way I want and not having to pay the consequences for someone else's bad choices," she shares in *AARP.*[49]

So, if you're at that point, or sliding toward it, you're most likely facing the biggest fear thrust upon childfree and childless women, a twist on the "die-alone" scenario—who will you have to take care of you as you age? Caregiving is a concern for everyone, even happily coupled people because, as we've already discussed, romantic partners sometimes die or become disabled or ill first, forcing women into the role of caregiver or widow. Figuring out what kind of caregiving we may need and want and who will do it is something all of us need to think about and plan for. According to the Institute on Aging, 19 percent of women between ages sixty-five and seventy-four need help with at least one self-care activity; that jumps to 53 percent for women age eighty-five and older.[50]

And that includes moms. Let's be real—there is no guarantee that your child or children will be willing or able to care for you, even if you hope they will or attempt to bribe them. With the rise in divorce and multiple marriages, your children's time and energy may be taxed by trying to care for your former spouse, and whatever step-parents and even multiple stepparents that might be part of their extended family, including in-laws if they're married, while they may be caring for their own children or an ill or disabled partner. And there's a fair number of parents who are estranged from their adult children.[51]

In other words, just the fact that you have a child or children does not guarantee you a caregiver when you need or want one.

Mothers can be just as clueless about planning for their aging future selves as childfree and childless women, notes Jody Day, founder of Gateway Women, a global friendship and support network for childless women, author of *Living the Life Unexpected: How to Find Hope, Meaning and a Fulfilling Future Without Children,* and childless by circumstance. Neither can truly afford to leave things to chance, but it's especially essential for older women without children.

"With social care systems around the world breaking down under the combined pressure of aging populations and neoliberal underinvestment, we can no longer rely on the state to be there for us. And it's not just intimate and residential care we need, it's advocacy; it's having a trusted younger person to help us manage the complex logistical and administrative tasks of modern living so that we can continue to age in place, if that's our wish. Many childless women have learned to be fiercely independent, particularly if they are also unpartnered, as many are. Developing connections with other younger childless women is going to be crucial to fill this need; it's not a quick fix, reciprocal trust doesn't form overnight and so it's vital to start building real social capital in those relationships long before you might want to rely on them," says Day, who is in her late fifties.[52]

We'll talk more about building and maintaining connections, community, and friendships—something women generally do well—in chapter 5. But let's get back to the narrative that women don't find a romantic partner later in life. Sometimes they do, and sometimes those partners come with children.

NEVER TOO LATE FOR LOVE

Vice President Kamala Harris was a never-married, childfree fifty-year-old woman when she married attorney Doug Emhoff, also fifty, in 2014, and instantly became stepmom—or "momala"—to his two children. And by all accounts, they have an equitable marriage, the kind that many women nowadays say they want but rarely end up having.[53]

Facebook chief operating officer Sheryl Sandberg, mom to two who was widowed at age forty-five, got engaged in 2020 at age fifty to a man four years younger than she is, Tom Bernthal, a father to three children.[54]

Celebrated author Anne Lamott, a mom to one son and a grandmother to one grandson, married for the first time at age sixty-five to a slightly younger man, Neal Allen, whom she met on an online dating site, and is dad to four adult children.[55]

All three of those attractive and accomplished men most likely could have dated and married women much younger than they are. We have seen this happen over and over, and research indicates that the older a man is when he marries, the more likely his wife will be younger — anywhere from seven to thirteen years younger — whether he's rich and educated or not.[56] That Emhoff, Bernthal, and Allen didn't skew younger just proves that confident, smart men have no problem committing to women their age or even older.

Look at France's President Emmanuel Macron and his wife, Brigitte Trogneux. There's a twenty-five-year age gap between them — she's the older one — and yet they seem to be in a marriage of equals. Same with the marriage between actor Aaron Taylor-Johnson and director Sam Taylor-Johnson, with a twenty-four-year age gap between them; Taylor-Johnson gave birth to their second child in 2012, when she was forty-four.

Neither Macron nor Taylor-Johnson seems to worry about what might happen as their much older wives get even older. Neither seems to be trapped by a narrow version of what a relationship *should* look like — and what their women *should* look like. And neither is letting society dictate what they know is right for them.

But we are so bombarded with images of older celebrity men dating and marrying women much younger than they are that it's easy to convince ourselves that no man around our age would want us. Clearly, that isn't the case. And let's face it — if a man our age isn't interested in dating a woman our age, well, he's probably not the kind of man we're interested in anyway. And that's OK.

For many women, especially Boomers, dating isn't even for marriage (Gen Xers are a bit more enthusiastic about saying, "I do").[57] Dating later in life is in many ways different from dating when you're young, when you may want a spouse and children. By the time women are in their forties, fifties, and beyond, many have full lives and while they might want to have someone around to do fun things with, and maybe have sex with, many believe they'll be fine whether they find a partner or not. In other words, dating is just to enhance whatever they already have.[58] It's similar for lesbian women, who aren't necessarily interested in starting long-term relationships at midlife either.[59]

So, when we hear that older women don't marry as often as older men, it would be easy to believe that the reason they don't is because they can't find someone to wed. That may indeed be true for some older women. For many more women, however, it's a choice. In fact, single women age fifty and older are much less likely than single men to say they'd tie the knot "if the right person came along."[60]

And if we gals are going to couple up, we're a lot more discriminating on things we may have been more generous about in our youth, particularly when it comes to attractiveness. Yes, we want a looker. Why not? The singles least likely to compromise on a potential partner's attractiveness were aged sixty and older, according to dating website Match.com's annual "Singles in America" survey. Survey adviser Helen Fisher, a biological anthropologist at the Kinsey Institute, suggests it may be because older women (and men) don't feel as pressured to find a romantic partner than they may have been when they were younger, especially if they were looking to have children.[61]

As many of the women Gail Sheehy interviewed for her book *Sex and the Seasoned Woman: Pursuing the Passionate Life* told her, "It is interesting that the most common phrase of defiance I hear in interviews with women who have divorced by midlife is, 'I don't want to defer anymore.' There is a double meaning: They don't want to defer to a husband's wishes just because he's the man. And they don't want to defer exploring their own dream until it dries up for good."[62]

But there are many older women who do want to wed again. My favorite later-in-life romantic stories happened to two of my girlfriends in wonderfully spontaneous ways.

When Leslie's son left for college, she transformed his bedroom in her San Francisco Bay Area house into an Airbnb guest room. Leslie had long been a single mom and, in her late forties, had pretty much given up on finding love. One day, a guy booked her room for three nights. They hit it off as soon as he walked through her door. Seven months later, she left her California home to live with him in Austin, Texas. They married in 2018 when she was fifty and he was fifty-seven.

Kathleen and Dan were neighbors in the San Francisco Bay Area when their children were young. Neither of their spouses was as enamored with the music of the Grateful Dead as they were, so the two Deadheads often went to Dead concerts together. Fast forward decades later and Kathleen is at the New Orleans Jazz Festival in 2015 with friends. Amid thousands of other festival goers, she spotted a familiar face—her old neighbor Dan. They chat, happy to reconnect, and discover both are now divorced. Months later, Dan moves to the Bay Area and in 2016, they wed, when she was fifty-eight and he was fifty-seven.

OK, those kinds of serendipitous meet-cutes are admittedly rare. Still, they bust the narrative that there's an expiration date for women to find love. I call BS.

EVEN LATER LOVE

After two marriages and divorces, Eve Pell did not expect to say "I do" again, and yet she did, when she was seventy-one and he was eighty-one. The San Francisco Bay Area residents, who met as part of a running group, couldn't help but wonder, "How lucky are we to find love late in life?"

They were hardly the only ones, as Pell discovered when she wrote a "Modern Love" column for the *New York Times* in 2013, two years after her husband died of cancer. Originally rejected, her column was among the most-read columns of all times and was even turned into an episode of the rom-com TV series based on the weekly columns.

After her column ran, Pell heard from hundreds of older people who had also found love late in life, and they were eager to share their stories with her. That became the basis of her 2015 book, *Love, Again: The Wisdom of Unexpected Romance.*

Age and all that comes with living a long life had in many ways prepared them for love, she told me. And without the distractions of growing careers and children, older people have the luxury of time to spend on each other.

"You know when you are getting together with this person, one of you is going to see the other die and you're willing to deal with that. The whole shadow of mortality gives an intensity and a bittersweetness to these late-in-life relationships that you don't have when you're younger," she tells me. "You've had your career, you've had your children, you have nothing left to do but love each other and be happy."[63]

That sounds incredibly sweet.

Eve, now in her mid-eighties, has had a new partner for the past few years. Love, again, indeed.

THE HARD STUFF

This is not to say that all who are seeking a romantic partner at midlife or later can always easily find one.

Dating can be challenging for women with disabilities. They tend to date later in life and marry much less than abled-bodied women, but it certainly isn't impossible.[64] Robin Wilson-Beattie, a quadriplegic whom we met in chapter 2, married for the second time in 2017. She and her husband are polyamorous, and she delights in busting any preconceived notions people may have about disabled women having more than one sexual partner at a time.[65]

For Black women, who are the least likely to marry and remain married and if they do wed, it's later than White and Hispanic women,[66] dating at midlife is hard, sociologist Cheryl Y. Judice discovered while doing research for her book, *Interracial Relationships Between Black Women and White Men.* Which is why she encourages Black women to date and marry White men, despite having a history of being enslaved by them. It makes those relationships "the most different, the most daring."[67]

It also can be challenging for older lesbians, Paige Averett, a North Carolina State University professor who researches LGBTQ and minorities issues, tells me.[68] Although many used to frequent lesbian bars to meet potential romantic partners and find community, hanging around bars often doesn't seem all that attractive as one ages (and the pandemic shut down many bars for a long time, forcing many to close permanently). Plus, many lesbians often feel a need to go back in the closet as they age for fear of discrimination, making finding new potential partners a challenge. Many Boomer lesbian women were teens when the gay rights movement came to the national consciousness in the late 1960s, and so they came of age in an environment that was far less accepting and much more stigmatizing than lesbian teens experience today. That may influence their self-image and their attitudes about forming romantic relationships.

Increasingly, going online or on dating apps is the way women look for love; 9 percent of those aged fifty to sixty-four say they've tried it. But if you're anything like my single sixty-something gal friends, you are not swiping right on the idea. They've either deleted their profiles long ago or allow it to frustrate them for a few months until they give up on it, only to go back online eventually and then give up again. Online dating can be frustrating and doesn't always lead to dates, let alone mates.

In his 2017 study of dating apps, Stanford University sociologist Michael Rosenfeld discovered that more than 80 percent of single heterosexual men and women had not gone on any dates in the past year.[69] And while 20 percent of single hetero women who met at least one guy for dating or sex at age forty, just 5 percent did at age sixty-five. That sounds sobering but remember—many older women see dating as a way to enhance whatever they already have. There's no reason to meet IRL if, after a few texts back and forth or a phone call or two, the guy's just not all that.

Given that, it may be surprising to learn that lesbian women and middle-aged hetero women are actually meeting mates online— Anne Lamott is just one example. And while I haven't met a "forever" mate on dating sites and apps, I have met quite a few I have enjoyed time with, including one I dated for nearly six years.

In fact, Rosenfeld found that online dating is the predominant way same-sex people meet and couple up.[70]

One thing that can make online dating harder for women age fifty and older is the digital divide. Access is a problem, particularly for women who are disadvantaged, whether socioculturally, economically, or physically.[71] No internet, no online dating. But there are always other ways to find what we're looking for.

No matter what you're seeking at this stage of your life, here's an interesting discovery to ponder: an international team of researchers surveyed more than 7,000 people from twenty-seven countries about what drives them, and contrary to a long-held popular belief, it isn't the search for "The One"—a romantic or sexual partner. Looking for a romantic partner—known as mate seeking—actually made people feel more anxious and depressed and less satisfied with their life. Anyone who has ever sought romantic love knows just how exhausting that can be! The people who were most satisfied with their life were those tending to long-term relationships and caring for loved ones—children or family.[72] And since family comes in all sorts of shapes and forms nowadays, it seems like there are many ways we boost our life satisfaction—by caring for them.

When you think about it, we have been forming ideas about romantic love since we were small. Our parents modeled it; we observed it with our friends, relatives, neighbors; we've taken in all sorts of conflicting messages from all sorts of media for decades, and almost all of us have experienced it in all sorts of forms. Now, decades into our life, we are fully aware that whatever fantasies we may have had about romantic love when we were younger, whatever we observed about it in real life, and whatever we've actually experienced, our beliefs about it have no doubt changed, perhaps many times. Now we know things about it. Now we look back at how we believed, as Emma Watson did, that we must have a romantic partner by age thirty so we can get on with things and realize that's untrue. In fact, at our age, we realize just how many things we've been told about romantic love and aging aren't actually true—including the belief that women aren't desirable romantic partners past a certain age, and that there's something wrong if a woman has no desire for a romantic partner.

Now, that's the kind of narrative busting I could fall in love with.

THINGS TO THINK ABOUT

How important is romantic love to you?
Do you believe you are "too old" to find new love?
How have your beliefs about romantic love changed as you aged?
How satisfying is how you're experiencing romantic love now?
How do you want to experience romantic love moving forward?

4

✝

I Feel Bad About More Than Just My Neck

Women are beautiful when they're young, and not after. Men can still preserve their sex appeal well into old age. . . . Some men can maintain, if they embrace it . . . cragginess, weary masculinity. Women just get old and fat and wrinkly.

—Tracy Letts, August: Osage County[1]

At 50, I am incapable of loving a woman of 50. I find that too old. They are invisible. I prefer the body of young women, that's all.

—Yann Moix, French actor[2]

When the singer-songwriter I was eager to see walked on the stage at San Francisco's Masonic Auditorium, I gasped. I've loved her for decades and had several of her albums but had never seen her perform live. And, there she was in front of me, her long gray hair flowing, her face free from any discernable makeup or cosmetic procedure, wearing a dress that barely hid a thick midlife body.

"Wow," I thought to myself, "she looks so . . . *matronly*."

Whoa, did I just think that? What a horrifying thought! I quickly had to check in with myself. Why was that the first thing that came to mind? After all, she's a beautiful, talented, activist, philanthropic woman and, then fifty-four—seven years younger than I—looked exactly her age.

What's wrong with that?

Nothing.

The real question was, what was wrong with me?

Now, I know our brains are wired to size up people within a few seconds of seeing them, an evolutionary necessity that helped us determine if a stranger posed a threat to us. But after that, we can take control of our thoughts.

It wasn't the first time I had an ageist thought and it wasn't the last. I am not proud of this. And I am willing to bet that you have had similar thoughts, not just of beloved musicians or celebrities, but of women you see every day—your co-workers, your new neighbor who looks to be about your age and is always way more put together than you are whenever you run into each other, the cute barista who practically has your drink ready for you as soon as you enter the coffee shop, the two women sitting at the bar getting the bartender's full attention as well as the attractive man sitting next to them, or your newly divorced BFF who all of a sudden looks so damn glowy.

Someone looks her age or doesn't look her age; someone clearly has had work done or hasn't and perhaps "should"; someone who looks so hot and youthful that you feel diminished; someone who looks so bad that you pride yourself for not looking "that bad."

We gals are constantly comparing ourselves with our sisters around us and not for the most positive reasons. Sometimes, it's because we're figuring out whether we're more likely to land a new lover than she is; other times it's because we see them as a threat— she could attract and steal the lover we already have or the one we have our eyes on. Sometimes we feel diminished because someone's aging better than we are, or vice versa. It doesn't have to be like that, of course. We're less likely to worry about those scenarios if we feel pretty good about our own attractiveness.[3]

Wait—is that even a thing? Can it possibly be true that all we have to do is be chill with our beauty and body, and then we can go about our life as we please without constantly measuring ourselves against other women? Research says yes. Unfortunately, it isn't as easy as it seems, and it doesn't get easier as we age.

"As women, we live in a world that feels fully justified in judging and assessing our physical appearance and are encouraged to place much of our self-worth in how favorably we are 'scored' on a set of criteria we didn't create," writes Alexandra H. Solomon in her 2019 book *Taking Sexy Back: How to Own Your Sexuality and Create the Relationships You Want.*[4]

We didn't create the criteria, true, but we have bought into it, and all too often, we are the ones doing the judging and assessing of other women around our age to see how we're holding up in a never-ending effort to look anything but our age and better than the women around us.

To what end?

A lot of anxiety and perhaps even depression, evidently.

According to a recent *AARP* study, three in ten women admit that their biggest anxiety about getting older is their appearance.[5]

If I can be honest, I have had more than a few "What fresh hell is this?" moments looking in my mirror in the morning to know how true that is. Every day seems to bring a new assault on my go-to belief that I'm holding up OK for my age. It's not my biggest concern, though—staying healthy for as long as I can is my main concern. And yet for many women, the anxiety they feel over the loss of their attractiveness is greater than their fears about declining health as they age.[6] That anxiety gets in the way of their sex lives, which as we saw in chapter 2, actually matters to many older women.[7] And some say that anxiety may also put us at a greater risk of depression and other internalizing disorders.[8]

All because we live in a society that not only doesn't value a woman who looks her age, but that also convinces us that we can't be beautiful past a certain age—although we probably should spend a lot of time and money on products and procedures anyway to keep or enhance what little beauty we may have just in case. In other words, women just can't win.

Overwhelmingly, the messages women of all ages, but especially as the decades pass by, hear try to convince us that our bodies are problematic the way they are. We must do something to fix them before it's too late.

What if we got different messages? What if the beauty of older women, especially older women of all sizes, abilities, colors, sexualities, was a given in the media? What if we saw, read about, and experienced more than images of thin, young, White, hetero, abled women? What would we do differently? Would the loss of attractiveness as we age cause us less anxiety? Would we celebrate ourselves "as is"? Would we feel more comfortable in our own skin? Would we have more time and energy to spend on things other than our perceived deficiencies? And, as importantly, would we be more accepting of other women whose sizes, abilities, colors, gender identity, sexual orientation, and attractiveness differ from ours? The belief that "women are beautiful when they're young, and not after," as playwright Tracy Letts's character Violet—at sixty-five, she's a Boomer—says in her Pulitzer Prize-winning play actually causes women and girls real harm. Society's constant emphasis on women's physical attractiveness is a type of "beauty sickness," observes Renee Engeln, Northwestern University psychology professor and founder of the Body and Media Lab.

It's "what happens when women's emotional energy gets so bound up with what they see in the mirror that it becomes harder for them to see other aspects of their lives," she writes in her 2017 book *Beauty Sick: How the Cultural Obsession with Appearance Hurts Girls and Women.* "At a practical level, beauty sickness steals women's time, energy, and money, moving us further away from the people we want to be and the lives we want to live."[9]

PUTTING ON OUR BEST FACE

"Bring me my face cream," my mom called to me from her bed.

She was using a drugstore face cream by that point, a switch for her after many years as a cosmetologist selling high-end anti-aging cosmetics at an exclusive South Florida salon and spa.

It wasn't labeled an anti-aging cream—we'd already entered the cosmetic era promising "rejuvenation" and it had some scientific-sounding numbers and terms—but the irony did not escape me. My mom had just turned eighty-one and was in a rehab hospital in Ohio recuperating from her second open-heart surgery. Rejuvenation didn't seem to be on the agenda.

I brought her the face cream, watched her carefully smooth it on and rub it in as I had seen her do since I was a child, kissed her goodnight, and said goodbye—I was flying back home to the San Francisco Bay Area the next morning. Two days later, the hospital called; she had passed away in her sleep. She was still a beautiful woman, but clearly all those years of slathering on anti-aging creams did not stop her from aging or from developing wrinkles and age spots along the way.

"Live fast, die young and have a good-looking corpse," Willard Motley wrote in his 1947 novel *Knock On Any Door*, a quote that has wrongly been attributed to James Dean. If you don't want to die young, you probably won't have a good-looking corpse. Does that really matter?

In 2017, *Allure* magazine created controversy when it proclaimed that it was banning the term "anti-aging" from its pages because it sent the wrong message, the editor-in-chief announced, a message that "aging is a condition we need to battle."[10] But, as many have noted, that just forced cosmetic companies to use other terms— "regeneration," "renewal," "radiance," "glow," "luminosity," etc.— to convince women that their products will maintain our youth and beauty.[11] At some point, cosmeceuticals—a mash-up of "cosmetics" and "pharmaceuticals"—became popular, promoting not just beauty but also (mostly unfounded) medical benefits.[12]

"There's a wellness factor now," L'Oréal Paris global makeup director Val Garland says. "It isn't just makeup—it's about nurturing the skin."[13] As if concealer or bronzer could somehow make you "well."

Perhaps inspired by *Allure*'s decision, the Royal Society for Public Health, the world's oldest public health body, according to its website, issued a statement a year later recommending, among other things, that the cosmetics and beauty industries abandon the use of the term anti-aging forever, calling it ageist. Instead, they suggest, why not feature older people in all sorts of media so wrinkles, dark spots, and other visible signs of aging will be seen as "normal."[14] It's just what aging skin looks like, and there's nothing horrible about it or anything to fear. And, in fact, all of us probably love, respect, and treasure people whose skin looks like that. I did and still do; my grandparents when they were alive, my parents as they aged, and now my dear friends.

Still, I am not immune to the messages. I struggle to accept my aging skin, and so I slather my face with rose hip and black seed serum, probiotic and vitamin C day cream, and ultra-hydrating antioxidant night cream every day, and sunscreen when I go outside. The brand doesn't matter to me; I read the labels and avoid any product with toxic ingredients, which many have and certainly will not offer any sense of "wellness."

But I do not delude myself. Like my beautiful mother, I can't buy myself out of aging, and neither can you.

And why would we even want to?

I remember shopping at a department store many years ago, when I was in my late forties, that offered a birthday discount. "Happy birthday," the cashier said to me cheerfully as she rang up my purchases, a woman who seemed to have quite a few years on me. "Thank you, but I can stop having them now," I said, half-jokingly. "No," she gently chided me. "You want to keep having birthdays."

She was right. I do, at least for a few more decades. I'm not done yet. I don't really want to be anti-aging; I want to age—aging means we're still alive, and that is a privilege not everyone gets to experience. Do I want to look as good as I can as I age? Hell yes, within reason. Meaning, I'm not interested in going under the knife or injecting myself with goodness knows what to look good.

And that opens up a huge divide for women—those who do and those who don't. Undergo cosmetic surgery, that is.

DOES SHE OR DOESN'T SHE?

While promoting her skincare line in 2021, JLo Beauty—it offers no promise of anti-aging, just the now popular substitute term "glow"—Jennifer Lopez found herself on the defensive when an Instagram follower accused her of using Botox. Nope, she wrote. No Botox, no injectables, no surgery, just "#beautyfromtheinsideout" and "#beautyhasnoexpirationdate."[15]

That's part of the problem—any woman who looks great naturally because of good genes or a life spent out of the sun or whatever reason, including just plain luck, is assumed to be doing something. Because so many women actually are doing something, or many things.

It probably won't be surprising for you to discover that women make up 92 percent of all cosmetic procedures, surgically and minimally invasive, according to the American Association of Plastic Surgeons. Considering $16.5 billion was spent on cosmetic procedures in the United States in 2018, women are almost single-handily keeping the industry alive. Well, not all women—non-Hispanic White women. They account for more than 12 million procedures, whereas Hispanics have a mere 1.9 million procedures followed by African Americans, 1.6 million, and Asian Americans, 1.2 million.

And the vast majority—49 percent—are between forty and fifty-five years old; women fifty-five and older account for the next largest group, at 26 percent.[16] That is no doubt because in the United States, a certain look is considered the epitome of beauty—thin, "fair" White skin, blue eyes, and long, straight blond hair.

In her book *Plucked: A History of Hair Removal*, Professor Rebecca Herzig lays out the dangerous extremes women have gone to in an effort to fit into societal norms, in this case their "unsightly" hair (unsightly to whom?).

Many women continued to go to X-ray epilation clinics to be smooth-skinned even when radiation was proven to be harmful and dangerous, giving many of the women lesions and cancer, and leading a few to death. Most women nowadays who laser, wax, shave, and thread away their body and facial hair describe their choices as "self-enhancement" and not societal pressure—they believe only other people, Herzig amusingly points out, "are dupes of social pressure, while narrating their (our) own actions as self-directed and free."[17]

I stand guilty. I shave my legs and underarms, I've waxed my lady parts (mostly for the pleasure of my lovers), I even threaded my eyebrows once. Then I microbladed my eyebrows, because sometimes we actually *do* want hair.

I don't fault or judge anyone for choosing to get cosmetic surgery, Botox, or any of the other procedures available to make us look younger. It's just not anything I want to do, and I am in awe of high-profile women who feel the way I do, not that there are many of them.

Actor Justine Bateman is one. After getting a lot of flack for having a face that was "looking old" when she was in her forties, she decided to push back and do . . . nothing. "I hated the idea that half the population was perhaps spending the entire second half of their lives ashamed and apologetic that their faces had aged naturally," she writes in her 2021 book *Face: One Square Foot of Skin*.[18]

I hear you, Justine.

Appearing on NPR's "Fresh Air" in 2018, two weeks before her sixtieth birthday, actor Annette Bening told host Terry Gross that she's not interested in getting work done—and here's the surprise—because she wants to continue to act. This seems at complete odds with Hollywood and its long-standing obsession with youth—especially for women. "I don't consider it virtuous—it's just me. That's my approach," she said. "I wanted to try to portray the age that I was and not get stuck in any given period of life."[19]

"Not get stuck in any given period of life," presumably younger if she had work done to make her look younger than her age. I had never heard that before, especially from someone in the spotlight. I've heard many older women say they wish they were younger—happily, many say they wouldn't want to go back to their twenties but their thirties seems to be the sweet spot[20]—and certainly many women seek cosmetic enhancements to look younger than they are. So, it was refreshing to hear an almost sixty-year-old woman say she's more than OK with looking like an almost sixty-year-old woman, especially in Hollywood, an industry that tends to ignore women past age forty and portrays women fifty and older in the worst possible ways, from frumpy to sickly.[21]

In her early sixties, actor Frances McDormand is a lot less generous toward the cosmetic surgery trend and a lot more vocal against it.

"Getting older and adjusting to all the things that biologically happen to you is not easy to do, and is a constant struggle and adjustment. So anything that makes that harder and more difficult—because I don't believe that cosmetic enhancement makes it easier; I think it makes it harder. I think it makes it much more difficult to accept getting older. I want to be revered. I want to be an elder; I want to be an elderess," she says.[22]

"My position has always been that the way people age and the signs that we show of aging is nature's way of tattooing. It's natural scarification, and the life you lead gives you the symbols and the emblems of your life, the road map you followed."[23]

Not only does McDormand reject the trend—no Botox, no fillers, no hair dye—she boldly appeared at the 2018 Academy Awards, where she won an Oscar for *Three Billboards Outside Ebbing, Missouri*, wearing no makeup, which is exceptionally daring for many women at the supermarket or the office, let alone Hollywood.

Are women missing an opportunity to control the narrative of aging however damn well we please by not celebrating women like Bateman, Bening, and McDormand?

Many of us dabbled in the "natural look" during the coronavirus pandemic. We basically had no choice.

The months of stay-home orders sent millions of women like me into uncharted beauty territory. We couldn't go to our hairdresser, or get a mani/pedi, or hit the weekly yoga class, or re-up the Botox, or have our eyebrows microbladed, or dye our eyelashes, or have our face exfoliated, or have our lady parts waxed.

In other words, we were unable to attend to all the beauty routines we've been told are essential to be our best self.

It was a time of Beauty, Interrupted, but whose version of beauty? Karen Karbo's book *Yeah, No. Not Happening: How I Found Happiness Swearing Off Self-Improvement and Saying F*ck It All—and How You Can Too* isn't the first book on the beauty industry—Naomi Wolf's *The Beauty Myth: How Images of Beauty Are Used Against Women* set the stage in 1991—but it's the latest to make it pretty clear that consumer culture has made huge profits by convincing us that we aren't "all that" on our own, but if we just bought product A, B, and C and did X, Y, and Z, we might finally be our best selves. Until, of course, they find another thing we need to improve, and that can only be improved by purchasing something.

Even during the pandemic, when some of us were lucky enough to work from home or others were unemployed at home, we were still being sold products to "embrace the natural look" while in quarantine.[24] Couldn't the natural look mean whatever you look like naturally?

Many women walked around sporting grombre locks—gray, white, or silver roots slowly overtaking the dyed hair at the ends. Some women embraced the look, others struggled. Podcast host/creator and author Manoush Zomorodi struggled with it at first. In an unfortunately titled article, "A Self-Indulgent Ode to Old Lady Hair," Zomorodi slowly begins to accept her new look, feeling a need to be a public woman with gray hair.

It was a love/hate thing for her, but others did not share her potential love. "Growing out your hair will make you look old. Don't do it," a seventy-year-old male neighbor tells her. (Wish we could see the visuals on him: Bald? Gray? Toupee? Comb over?) Her ten-year-old daughter also isn't a fan—"'I don't want an old mommy,' she told me. Her comments hurt my feelings, but I also kind of understood that my transformation was, well, shocking. . . . Within months, I'd gone from passing for thirty-seven years old (or so I've been told) to looking my forty-seven years. It's disconcerting for both of us."[25]

An "old mommy." At forty-seven! Where is a ten-year-old learning what a mommy looks like? Not just the media, obviously—if you're an "older" mom who shows up at school events, your child will be aware of whether you look young or don't compared to the other moms, no matter your age.

But gray hair isn't "old lady hair." Women can turn gray in their twenties, although just a fraction of 1 percent between the ages of twenty-five to thirty-four are completely silver, according to an Australian study. But 25 percent of men and women between the ages of twenty-five to thirty-four had some graying, and more than 60 percent had gray hairs between ages thirty-five and forty-four.[26]

After age forty-five, well, things get real with hair color. That said, there's a new generation of young women embracing their gray locks. More than 223,000[27] women follow the @grombre Instagram account, many who share their stories and support each other. Interestingly, one woman was shocked to discover that women were giving her a harder time about going gray than the men were.[28]

We didn't always. Something has happened to women since the days of *The Golden Girls,* the beloved sitcom that revolved around four women who lived together, three of whom were in their fifties and one in her eighties. It's interesting to observe what was acceptable for fifty-something women to look like in the 1980s, when the show started, and what's OK now. At fifty-one, Rue McClanahan was the youngest cast member who also happened to play the part of the youngest character, Blanche, who was fifty-three. Bea Arthur and Betty White were both sixty-three at the time and played characters in their fifties. Both also happened to be fully gray.[29]

The Golden Girls showed us that it was OK if women in their fifties had gray hair.

A few of my sixty-something girlfriends no longer dye their hair and look radiant with their silver manes. I barely have gray hair, just some frizzy action around my ears that my friends tease me about, and a lot of mousey brown—my parents grayed very late—and so I am not there yet.

But I lived for months without having my hair highlighted or cut, and not putting anything on my face but whatever creams and serums I had in my bathroom cabinet, unable to visit my usual beauty shops and fearful about having too many packages delivered before science indicated the virus was spreadable through the air, not surfaces. I made it through the lockdown just fine, although I will admit that getting that first haircut and, yes, highlights, was highly satisfying.

But, what I and many women learned during the lockdown was that we were still likeable, loveable, a valued employee, and, yes, even fuckable, "as is."

Clearly, Lopez doesn't "need" cosmetic surgery to fit into the beauty standard—she *is* the beauty standard, or the idealized beauty standard—so it's easy for her to reject it. Still, on her cosmetic line website, she is pretty clear that beauty products, even hers, are not enough to keep women looking good at any age, aka #beauty hasnoexpirationdate. Her beauty regimen involves more than just creams, face masks, and serums—it's about getting eight hours of sleep, taking supplements, applying sunscreen, and living what she considers a healthy lifestyle: no booze, no smoking, eating good food, exercising, and hydrating.

There's a lot of science around some of that—especially using sunscreen, getting sleep, and exercising—and we'd be smart to put more energy into those very doable and generally inexpensive activities. But it's a lot easier to sell women on procedures and cosmetics to deal with the damage that things like years of exposure to the sun, booze, smoking, eating processed food, lack of sleep, and inactivity will bring on. Lest we forget, there's a lot of money to be made on pushing supplements, health food, exercise, and even bottled water, "artisanal" or not.

In her study of the ageist language in ads for cosmetics, Justine Coupland, a senior lecturer at Cardiff University in Wales asks, "How can advertisers persuade women that stopping the ageing process or, rather, disguising its effects on the body is achievable?" It's easy, she says, if you not only make aging skin seem pathological, but also lay on some guilt by making women feel "responsible" for their wrinkles.[30]

But even if we follow Lopez's routine, we still won't look like her (sorry!). And not every woman has the luxury of avoiding working in the sun, or the time or ability to exercise or have eight hours of sleep, or the financial means to eat well or buy sunscreen or has easy access to drinkable water. That shouldn't exclude them from living Lopez's #beautyfromtheinsideout—right?

Not necessarily.

WHOSE BODY MATTERS?

"We did not start life in a negative partnership with our bodies," writes activist and poet Sonya Renee Taylor in her book *The Body Is Not an Apology*.[31] Regardless, she notes, "those of us who do not believe we have the 'right body' spend decades of our life and dollars trying to shrink, tuck, and tame ourselves into the right body all the while forfeiting precious space on the planet because we don't feel entitled to it."[32]

Those who nip and tuck shouldn't be dissed, however, says Sesali Bowen—@BadFatBlackGirl on social media—author of a forthcoming book *Notes From a Trap Feminist: A Manifesto for the Bad Bitch Generation*. Black women who have spoken out against plastic surgery tend to fall into the conventionally attractive category, Bowen says. Like J.Lo, they don't "need" surgery. At the same time, they are judging women who feel pressured to attain unattainable beauty standards and policing how they choose to fit into those standards.

"Singling out plastic surgery as both unnecessary and unnatural is missing the bigger picture," she writes. "People with marginalized bodies are acutely aware of the consequences of not meeting the standards of physical beauty. Black women's bodies are constantly policed, targeted for violence, marked as deviant or excessive and mined for cultural appropriation. Fatphobia, transphobia, and ableism are part of our daily realities, especially for women of color."[33]

Despite that, the studies done on Black women's beauty and body image (and there are very few, sadly) indicate Black women generally are more satisfied with their body image. They're more accepting of larger bodies and don't fear having one; they aren't as obsessed with dieting; and—this seems key—they are less likely to internalize sociocultural standards of beauty than White women do.[34]

Even when midlife and older women fit the standards of physical beauty, however, they are scrutinized and judged.

When J.Lo and Shakira turned the Super Bowl 2020 halftime show into a display of fierce female power and unapologetic female sexuality—at fifty and forty-three years old respectively—many viewers were shocked and upset, prompting more than 1,300 complaints to the Federal Communications Commission. Some found their performance pornographic and not "family friendly," whatever that means. But some women had a more inward-focused reaction along the lines of middle-aged author Jennifer Weiner: *Oh, do I have to look like that at fifty, too?*

In an opinion piece in the *New York Times*, "I Feel Personally Judged by J.Lo's Body," Weiner writes of Lopez, "Some members of my social-media community were in awe. Others—myself included—were feeling personally judged. I'm just a few months younger than J.Lo, and, with every birthday, I have asked: Is this the year it ends? . . . Women watch a fifteen-minute show featuring elite entertainers and, in some cases, end up feeling bad about ourselves. . . . Women see inspiration or goals we've failed to attain or a pretty stick to beat ourselves up with. We hear a voice (sponsored by Weight Watchers and Revlon and Planet Fitness and Jenny Craig) whispering, 'This can be yours, if you just work hard enough.'"

Weiner admits that she would rather happily wrap herself in her Eileen Fisher tunic and bifocals, and embrace turning fifty "as the year when I'd be done."[35]

"Done" is an interesting word to describe what she's feeling, and can be interpreted many ways. Done with what? Is she channeling Nora and Delia Ephron's famous line from their Off-Broadway show, "Love, Loss, and What I Wore"—"When you start wearing Eileen Fisher, you might as well say, 'I give up'."

What Weiner seems to be saying is that she'd like to be done with seeking the male gaze and thus, having to primp, dye, Botox, wax, diet, and exercise to compete with other women for that gaze at an age when society tells us we're invisible anyway, so why even bother?

Maybe you can relate to her desire to be "done" and also are gravitating toward cozier and more forgiving clothing, going gray, not wearing makeup (and during the pandemic, many embraced that look). Still, I wonder why isn't there room to celebrate or champion—or at least not feel diminished by—women who don't want to be done, who want to work on themselves, however hard and in whatever way, because that's when they feel their best? Why do we have to "beat ourselves up" or feel bad about ourselves if other older women are breaking barriers?

In fact, we don't always do that.

There weren't similar outcries when fashion designers started having women in their fifties and older women walk the runways during fashion weeks in recent years. No, we celebrated that. Finally, we collectively sighed, older women are visible.[36]

Or when Forbes introduced a "50 Over 50" list for the first time in 2020, dedicated to women "who have achieved significant success later in life," such as Speaker Nancy Pelosi, in her eighties; and Christine Lagarde, president of the European Central Bank, and Ursula von der Leyen, the European Commission president, both in their sixties.

Or when six midlife and older women — Amy Klobuchar, Elizabeth Warren, Kamala Harris, Kirsten Gillibrand, Tulsi Gabbard, and Marianne Williamson — ran in the 2020 Democratic presidential race.

We didn't feel "personally judged" by any of them. No, we celebrated and championed their achievements, especially when Harris, at age fifty-six, became America's first female vice president. So, it seems that the only time we judge women is when they look better than we think we do and we believe they are somehow using their beauty — or "flaunting" it — to gain some sort of an advantage.

Model Paulina Porizkova wasn't seeking to gain an advantage when posting a nude photo of herself on Instagram in 2021, when she was fifty-five. Was she flaunting it? Inspiring other women? Making them feel bad about themselves (as if all of us could come close to looking like her at any age!)? What she got was a lot of criticism. Her response was spot-on:

"When I was in my twenties and thirties, the less I wore — the more popular I was. In my forties, I could walk around practically naked and illicit (sic) nothing more than a ticket for public indecency. At fifty, I am reviled for it. 'Put on your clothes, grandma. Hungry for attention, are you? A little desperate here? You're pathetic.' Why is sexiness and nudity applauded in a woman's youth and reviled in her maturity? Because of men."[37]

Consumer culture and male-dominated media have no problem exploiting women's bodies and beauty to sell stuff, even if the models are older (Isabella Rossellini is once again the face of Lancôme after being dumped by the cosmetic company at age forty-three for being too old); why can't women take control of the narrative and celebrate our beauty and body publicly the way we want to?

"People can get confused when women use their sexuality and wisdom. When it comes to power, it's often either/or," observes psychology professor Wendy Walsh.[38]

Here's the sad truth — attractive women actually do have an advantage, whether they "flaunt" it or not. They are perceived to be healthier, smarter, more likeable, and more trustworthy, and can use their good genes to get ahead in work and find a prime romantic partner. And if they are involved in politics, they get more votes, too.[39]

What are we to do about beautiful older women who "flaunt" their looks? Spend our limited time and energy on Earth being envious of them or judging while putting ourselves down?

Why can't we celebrate women for all of what we are, brains and beauty, and, yes, sexuality, as we age?

THAT DAMN MALE GAZE

The many beauty routines hetero women often indulge in to fit into a narrow version of what's considered beautiful is a way to not only be worthy of the "male gaze," but also to perhaps be feminine enough to get the ultimate prize—a man of our own. It also sets us up to constantly compete with other women, thus disrupting friendships (more on that in chapter 5).

I remember walking into a local restaurant with a girlfriend years ago, both of us in our early fifties and a few years out of our divorces and seeing a sea of beautiful single women about a decade younger seated at the bar with the same hopes we had, of meeting an attractive age-appropriate man, or at least having a fun evening of flirting with one or two. We looked at each other—*we're not going to be able to compete with that,* we simultaneously thought—walked out, and headed in search of another restaurant where we might have better luck.

It seems silly now, especially in light of what Cindy Gallop, whom we met in the Introduction, told me. Not about beauty per se, but addressing the way hetero women often rely on it to capture a man's attention and, if we're lucky, affection, and how it forces us to constantly compare ourselves with other women, which seems to become more urgent as we age. "One of the best moments of my life was the day I stopped looking for 'The One.' As girls we grow up being told that our entire life is the search for 'The One.' In our teens and twenties, every social event we go to (we think), 'Will he be there?' . . . This dynamic forces us to compete with other women, which I don't want, and at some point in my early thirties, I said, fuck this. Oh my god, the liberation. I could just go to social events and enjoy myself."[40]

Going out with no agenda other than enjoying myself either solo or with friends is exactly where my head's at now, in my sixties. I'm working on accepting my aging body and face, but I'm right there with Frances McDormand—it's a "constant struggle and adjustment."

"Consider all the times you have assessed your value or lack thereof by comparing yourself to someone else. When we are saddled with body shame, we see other bodies as things to covet or judge," Taylor writes.[41] "We think tons of repugnant, petrifying, miserable things about our own bodies and other folks' bodies every single day."[42]

As I did with my beloved singer-songwriter. I truly owe her an apology.

Jennifer Burgmann was not quite ready to give up the male gaze, although she is married (and I think a lot of married women can relate). She was considered pretty by societal standards until age thirty-eight, when she became disabled and needed a wheelchair after surviving a life-threatening illness. For the past ten years, she has had to come to peace with her crooked body, she writes in a post titled "I'm Disabled, Middle-Aged, Menopausal—and Beautiful" on *The Mighty*, an online community for people facing health challenges.

"Men rarely look at me with romantic interest, if they even notice me at all. In the decade since being disabled, I have been flirted with only one time, and asked out on a date once. (I am happily married, so it was a 'no,' but it's still nice to know you are considered attractive.) This severely affected my body image and self-esteem. I was not accustomed to being discounted or rejected because of my appearance, and it hurt," she writes.

But as she hit menopausal age and adapted to her body's limitations while appreciating what it still could offer her, she discovered that "physical appearance is the least important aspect of beauty."

I thought about what the late actor Helen McCrory wrote. When she portrayed Leo Tolstoy's great heroine, Anna Karenina, in the British television series of the same name at age thirty-one, McCrory was unfavorably compared to Greta Garbo, who played Anna in 1935, when she was thirty. As Tolstoy wrote her, Anna was no beauty. But, then again, Anna and other women of her era didn't have to compare themselves with images on social media.

"Anna's appeal lies in the visceral rather than the physical," McCrory wrote in *The Guardian*. "Today, women are constantly made aware of the physical impression they create; sexuality is defined by the male view of it and women's sexual role is seen as passive and usable. The images of women's bodies that appear in advertising and in the media signal vulnerability, needing to be saved and being sexually available at all times. At least Anna and her contemporaries escaped this."[43]

I would not want to go back to Anna's days, when women had to marry to survive and were basically confined to the home, but there's a lot to be said about not having women's looks and sexuality being defined by men, ads, and social media.

As a fifty-year-old trans woman told me, "On the one hand I didn't grow up with the pressure women face over appearance every minute. But on the other that meant that when I did transition, I was dumped into the deep end of those expectations with little fanfare. I had thought, while I was presenting as male, that I kinda got it, but it was still a shock to be so immediately yoked to my appearance."[44]

The thing is, many women are like Jennifer Burgmann—aware that they are being objectified by men, making it easy for them to also start seeing themselves as an object. And when that happens, they can't help but notice when they're no longer turning heads, says New York psychologist Alison Carper. "As humans, we all need to be recognized, but as we grow older, the manner of recognition we search for can change. A subject is someone who experiences her own agency, who is aware of how she can and does have an impact on others and how she is, ultimately, the author of her own life. She is aware of the responsibility this carries."[45] In other words, we can orchestrate what's turning heads, like "the visceral rather than the physical."

Obviously, there is no desire for the male gaze from lesbian women so they often don't have quite the same kind of anxiety about the physical signs of aging as hetero women do.[46] In fact, midlife often comes as a great relief for many lesbians, LGBTQ researcher Dr. Paige Averett tells me, mostly because it finally frees them of any unwanted gazing by men who wrongly assume—as men too often do—that they're interested in them.[47]

Many lesbians also don't seem to buy in to the cultural obsession on youth, thinness, and beauty as much as hetero and bisexual women do, but they're not immune to it either.[48] That said, they don't let it get in the way of other things, like sex.[49] If you're not feeling good in your own skin, it's going to interfere with your sexual pleasure, as we discussed in chapter 2, and life satisfaction in general.

Which means that there is a huge swath of people—hetero and bisexual women, as well as gay men—who are trying to fit into what men consider attractive, which is generally pretty narrow, and then suffering if we don't.

Why have we given them all that power?

We don't have to. I'm enamored of the women throughout history who owned their own power (no need to be "empowered," a word I have come to hate when it relates to women when we clearly have our own power). As profiled in historian Betsey Prioleau's 2003 book *Seductress: Women Who Ravished the World and Their Lost Art of Love,* some women were nowhere near what society would consider beautiful or even attractive, but they were strong, sexy, and accomplished women nevertheless. And—my favorite part—they had the gifts of charm and wit.

"They teach women they don't have to cave in to traditional femininity. Better still, they don't have to be beautiful or young, hold their tongues, play tricks, or teeter on Manolo Blahniks to captivate men," Prioleau explains in an interview. "The seductress's biggest lesson is the importance of cerebral lures. The most powerful mental charm was, and is, the allure of a big, forever-interesting person. That's the best news for 21st century women."[50]

If only twenty-first-century women were truly listening.

"YOU LOOK GREAT!"

Back when my marriage was imploding, I couldn't sleep and I couldn't eat. So, of course, I lost weight. I didn't have a heck of a lot to lose, but I shed about eight pounds pretty quickly. I got down to about what I weighed in high school—when I was convinced that I was fat.

As much as my friends were concerned about me, here's what I heard from them as well as from acquaintances: "You look great!"

Hey, thanks. My life is falling apart but at least I look good!

This happened to many of my girlfriends as well, all of who, like me, got divorced in their late forties.

When we began to feel more comfortable navigating our life as new divorcees, we embraced our new skinnier bodies thanks to our Divorce Diets and kept the weight off—joking that it was nature's way to make us more attractive to whoever we imagined would be our next lovers.

It really isn't something to joke about. Women who lose weight at midlife could suffer problems when they're older, including poor physical function, and an increased risk of hip fractures and even death, new research indicates.[51]

It can also be problematic in the moment. In 1988, when she was thirty-four, Oprah Winfrey had lost sixty-seven pounds and dropped down to 145 pounds—her thinnest weight ever. She looked great. But Oprah admits her body was out of whack. Now she weighs more, but she's healthier.[52] That matters.

Journalist Pamela Druckerman experienced something akin to the Divorce Diet after being diagnosed with non-Hodgkin's lymphoma when she was in her early forties—something much scarier than a divorce, in my mind. No matter what she ate—huge bowls of pasta with cream sauce? Bring it!—she still lost weight, thanks to the chemotherapy she had to endure to tackle her cancer. This caused some of her female friends to be envious, she writes in her book *There Are No Grown-Ups: A Midlife Coming-of-Age Story.* "Getting ill is a crash course in other minds. I learn that . . . certain women will be jealous of how skinny you are, no matter what's causing it."[53]

I am so saddened and disturbed by that.

Druckerman has written extensively about how women have different lives in France—she has long lived in Paris with her husband and children—than women have in the States. And that includes a much healthier self-image.

"In America there's a lot of fat talk, where you're supposed to say negative things about your own body to the point where you can't even see yourself clearly. In France, even the women I know who don't have ideal proportions know what works on them. Women seem to understand what's attractive about them and know how to work it and own it and feel good about themselves. That feels culturally different."[54]

OK, so maybe you aren't French or don't live in France. Is there another way for you to feel good about your body? Sure—you could always become a nudist.

Stay with me.

Women who are nudists, meaning they go about doing what women do just without wearing clothes, tend to have a pretty healthy body image. Hanging around with other naked people whose bodies come in all shapes and sizes—but rarely the idealized images women believe we "should" look like—actually helps us feel better about our own body.[55]

That's what British photographer Amelia Allen discovered. For many years, she was immersed in the fashion world, photographing what would be considered "conventional beauty." But when she began taking photographs of naturalists, resulting in her book, *Naked Britain,* she realized how that industry presents a warped view of what's considered beautiful.

"Nudity demands that we look the person in the eye, to assess them for who they are, not what they project. Shorn of clothing, people must connect as equals, regardless of wealth, occupation or status," she says.[56]

Being naked in front of people you aren't having sex with opens you up to a different kind of vulnerability. V. Pendragon discovered that when she began living in a clothing-optional community in West Virginia twelve years ago. Although she only gets naked before others at the community's weekly dance parties, what she sees and what she's experienced as a woman in her mid-seventies and disabled by scleroderma, has been nothing but total acceptance by all around her.

"Here, it's like I don't even have crippled hands. There are so many variations of bodies and of ailments. We get people in wheelchairs, we have people with colostomy bags; you get all kinds of very visible maladies here. Nobody stares. Nobody would even dream of staring," shares Pendragon, who was a Playboy Bunny in her thirties. "Everybody is acutely aware of what it takes to be able to be naked in front of a bunch of people. Everybody in a place like this has said, I'm willing to be vulnerable, I'm willing to be open."[57]

I'll be honest. While I don't have any hang-ups walking around naked in front of my lovers and gal friends, doing that in front of neighbors, even close ones, is just not me. That said, I greatly appreciate that for some women, living *au naturel* helps them accept and embrace their aging body.

What would help you accept and embrace your aging face and body?

Some women fifty and older are doing that by deconstructing and defying gendered and ageist fashion and beauty standards by taking part in the "advanced style" movement, which got a huge boost from photographer Ari Seth Cohen in 2008 when he created the @advancedstyle Instagram account and a book and documentary about it.

Like the women we met in chapter 1 who used social media to bust the narratives about disability, misogynoir, childlessness, etc., women in their fifties and older have become Instagram influencers who use the platform to give a collective middle finger to gendered ageism in the fashion and beauty industries.[58]

Miniskirts? Bold colors? Tight clothes? Fishnets? Stilettos? Flashy jewelry? Who says women can't wear them past a certain age? Who says we're doomed to having to cover ourselves with the shapeless, black, white, and beige clothing that's so often seen as more appropriate for older women, even if it announces, as the Ephron sisters observe, that they've "given up?"

Can we at midlife and later in life learn to know what's attractive about ourselves and how to work it, as Druckerman says French women do? Can we change American culture? I think so. Look at what happened in China, where for centuries young girls' feet were bound so they wouldn't get larger than four inches, but ideally three inches—so-called "golden lotus" feet. Having tiny feet was a sign of status and beauty, and a form of eroticism for a potential husband's pleasure (although a new theory suggests it might actually have been for economic reasons).[59] But it wasn't men who broke their daughter's toes and arches —it was their mothers, grandmothers, and other older women.[60]

Foot binding stopped decades ago—it continued in some rural parts of China until the 1940s and the last factory making lotus shoes didn't shut down until 1999. Still, author Amanda Foreman notes, the practice continued for so long "in part because of women's emotional investment in the practice. The lotus shoe is a reminder that the history of women did not follow a straight line from misery to progress, nor is it merely a scroll of patriarchy writ large."[61]

Now young women in China are fast embracing Anglo-European images of beauty, for better or worse.[62] Importantly, it isn't for a potential romantic partner or husband's benefit; many women in China are delaying or rejecting marriage in a country with strict gendered roles.[63] Women have, slowly, changed society there.

I have now regained the eight pounds I lost from my Divorce Diet, and even added a few more during the pandemic. As much as I am not so happy about that extra weight and have begun to amp up my exercise routine, it has not stopped any man from dating me (as far as I know) or wanting to be sexual with me. Because it often doesn't bother someone who likes or loves us as much as it bothers us, as we saw in chapter 2 (not that everything has to be, or should be, about how the lovers in our life feel about us). Feeling bad about how our body looks interferes with our ability to feel sexual and enjoy sex, which then can lead to anxiety and depression, and, honestly, what is the good in any of that?[64]

As Naomi Wolf reminds us in *The Beauty Myth: How Images of Beauty Are Used Against Women*, "A culture fixated on female thinness is not an obsession about female beauty, but an obsession about female obedience. Dieting is the most potent political sedative in women's history; a quietly mad population is a tractable one."[65]

Again, I ask, why are we giving others that kind of power over us? Why do we do that to ourselves?

"One way to check if our desires for bodily change are motivated by authentic self-expression or shame is to ask ourselves, 'am I changing my body in ways that an oppressive body-shame system will reward me for?'" poet Taylor writes.[66]

Our faces and bodies are going to change as we age. This is normal. What's not normal, or what shouldn't be normal, is to feel shame about it and to harm ourselves in an effort to stop aging (which we can't). Foot binding continued because of "women's emotional investment in the practice." What beauty practices are you emotionally invested in, and for whose benefit?

THINGS TO THINK ABOUT

What are your biggest fears about your aging face and body? Why?
What messages have you heard and believe about older women's looks?
Are you changing the way you look to please others or yourself?
    Are you being influenced by what you see, or don't see, in media?
Do you assess your value by comparing yourself to other women?
Does how you feel about your face and body interfere with your pleasure, sexual and non-sexual?

5

From Mean Girls
to BFFs and Golden Girls

You can't sit with us!

—Gretchen Wieners, "Mean Girls"

When Rosalind Wiseman wrote her best-selling book *Queen Bees and Wannabes: Helping Your Daughter Survive Cliques, Gossip, Boyfriends, and the New Realities of Girl World* in 2002—a bestseller that inspired the hit movie and musical "Mean Girls"—she envisioned it as a guidebook for parents to help their daughters navigate their friendships.

It wasn't really about creating a "Kumbaya"-like sisterhood, although that is how it was often interpreted. It was more about giving girls tools to express their anger and disappointment about things between friends in a healthy way—directly, no meanness necessary. This matters because girls grow up to be women and expressing our anger directly is not what women are necessarily taught to do. And then we go from mean girls to mean grown-ups.[1]

"[S]trong women must be able to disagree with each other, otherwise, it comes across as if you're not strong enough and not competent enough to be able to disagree with each other, and that's total crap. If you're not used to being able to disagree and hold your own in a conversation, you sure as hell are not doing it in any other aspects of your life."[2]

Maybe this is what has inspired numerous books about how mean women are to other women, from *Mean Girls Grown Up: Adult Women Who Are Still Queen Bees, Middle Bees, and Afraid-to-Bees* to *Mean Girls, Meaner Women: Understanding Why Women Backstab, Betray, and Trash-Talk Each Other and How to Heal* to *In the Company of Women: Indirect Aggression Among Women: Why We Hurt Each Other and How to Stop.*

It would seem, then, that women, no matter how old we are, are just a bunch of bitches to each other. The narrative is that we're catty and we "compete, compare, undermine, and undercut" each another.[3] Evolutionary psychologists would say the reason why gals act that way is because we have no other choice. We're competing for the ultimate prize—a man. Well, not just *any* man—a man with the best genetic material to pass on to our offspring.[4] May the best woman win!

Clearly menopausal and postmenopausal hetero women are way past wanting a man for his genetic material, and lesbian women don't even give it much of a thought. So, what gives?

In some ways, it has nothing to do with men at all. According to psychologist Lynn Margolies, part of the problem is that women aren't expected to be competitive and aren't raised that way, so we can't use whatever natural edge we have in a healthy way. We also look to others to validate us. That creates what she says is a double bind that keeps us from achieving success. "Constrained by internal conflict and over-focus on others' reactions, many women endure the frustration of being unable to fulfill their true potential in terms of aggression, sexuality, and power."[5] And that can get in the way of our friendships with other women.

Yet how do we square that with perhaps the most beloved example of female friendship ever, the ones presented in *The Golden Girls*, the mid-1980s sitcom about four women, three fifty-somethings and one eighty-something, who share a house in Miami Beach, Florida? Although the last show aired in 1992, it is more popular now than when it first ran. Don't be surprised—there are good reasons why the show still resonates with women.

"What we built was a family," Tony Thomas, one of the executive producers, shares. "What we told America was life was not over just because you have an empty nest or you're divorced or your spouse died. You can create a new family and live another life. And I think the key to our show was the fact that life goes on. And there are other families. I think if you look at television, the most successful shows are shows that built within their cast a family that you loved to be with."[6]

Yes, yes, and yes. Life is not over at midlife, no matter what has happened before (and a big reason why I've written this book). And family can be much more than the narrow version we think it is — aka mom, dad, and kids. "Family" doesn't have to include anyone related to you by blood or marriage — it can be a "chosen family," a term coined by anthropologist Kath Weston in her book *Families We Choose: Lesbians, Gays, Kinship,* and one that has been embraced by the queer community.[7] And you can indeed live another life (but please, you do *not* have to reinvent yourself at midlife!).

Which is why *The Golden Girls* is also loved by so many LGBTQ people. "The gay community really felt these characters were an extension of their own communities," says Jeff Duteil, who wrote an episode of the show that included a lesbian crush. "They were accepting and funny and bitchy."[8]

Increasingly, older women are looking to re-create that kind of living arrangement with their girlfriends or even with strangers, according to sociologist Amy Blackstone.[9] It certainly seems more appealing than a lot of traditional options, including nursing homes.

In her 2015 book *How We Live Now: Redefining Home and Family in the 21st Century,* social scientist and singles advocate Bella DePaulo delves into *Golden Girls* arrangements as well as numerous other creative ways of living, often to foster friendships and community with just the right amount of sociability and solitude. Older people, especially older women, are among the most creative, she observes.[10]

Presumably, no woman is going to want to move in with bitches. Bitchy women who are accepting and funny? Sure. Just not out-and-out bitches.

Not to say that all was rosy all the time for the Golden Girls. Like any family, there was love and conflict, especially between Dorothy, played by Bea Arthur, and Blanche, played by Rue McClanahan. In some episodes, they cared for each other like the most loving, supportive sisters ever, and then the next week, they'd bicker and fight each other like, well, bitches. Still, the show highlighted female friends who were not mean girls — they could disagree with each other in healthy ways and work through it.[11]

But since *The Golden Girls,* there have been scant examples of media celebrating female friendship later in life. The only TV show that comes close is *Grace and Frankie,* featuring two seventy-something women who move in together after their husbands leave them for one another, and then slowly form a friendship despite starting off as frenemies. The Netflix series, which began in 2015, stars two longtime, real-life friends, Jane Fonda and Lily Tomlin.

The First Wives Club may be the last movie to celebrate female friendship later in life. It reunites three college friends, played by Goldie Hawn, Diane Keaton, and Bette Midler, all of whose husbands have left them, at midlife, for younger women. But *The First Wives Club* was made in 1996—a long time ago. And just like the women in *The Golden Girls* and *Grace and Frankie,* their status relates to men—they're either divorced or widowed.

WOMEN WITHOUT MEN

While we may not have the best media role models for female friendships, that doesn't mean they don't exist and that we can't have them—or that we don't need them. Because we do, especially as we age.

Sasha Roseneil, professor of interdisciplinary social science and dean of the faculty of social and historical sciences at University College London, suggests that female friendship "has historically been fundamental to feminist politics, identities and communities."[12]

Roseneil observes that Virginia Woolf's *A Room of One's Own* helped shape the work of twentieth-century feminists on the cultural neglect and devaluation of women's friendships—noting that the only way society had long seen women is though their relation with men. That is no longer the case, thankfully, but that doesn't mean it doesn't rear its ugly head from time to time.

Take the friendship of Oprah Winfrey and Gayle King, which started in 1976, when Oprah was twenty-two and Gayle was twenty-one, a decade before Oprah and Stedman Graham, her long-time romantic partner, began dating, and six years before Gayle got married. Oprah and Gayle have celebrated and supported each other ever since and have taken many vacations together; it's a friendship between two powerful and highly accomplished Black women based, they say, on honesty and trust.[13]

Still, as Oprah writes, "For years, people have marveled at our friendship—and sometimes misunderstood it. But anyone who has a soulful bond with a friend, a friend who would do anything for you, who revels in your happiness and is there to comfort you in your sadness, gets it exactly."[14]

What gets "misunderstood" is their closeness—it seems *too* close, especially for women who have romantic partners, although Gayle divorced in 1993. Surely, they must secretly be lesbians (as if that was some sort of a "bad" thing).[15]

The idea of who's having sex with whom and who isn't having sex is a source of confusion for people. Two female BFFs going on vacation without their romantic partners? They must be having sex! There's a tendency to sexualize all relationships, including same-sex relationships, notes author William Deresiewicz.[16]

"We have trouble, in our culture, with any love that isn't based on sex or blood. We understand romantic relationships, and we understand family, and that's about all we seem to understand," he writes. "We have trouble with mentorship, the asymmetric love of master and apprentice, professor and student, guide and guided; we have trouble with comradeship, the bond that comes from shared, intense work; and we have trouble with friendship, at least of the intimate kind. When we imagine those relationships, we seem to have to sexualize them."

Intimate friendships matter. One thing studies are pretty clear about is that social isolation and loneliness is bad for our health.[17] While many see marriage or romantic partnerships as the way out of that, many women outlive their romantic partners and a considerable amount of women still feel pretty lonely within those romantic partnerships, as we saw in chapter 3. So, it's no surprise that a number of married women say their friends are more important than their family in dealing with loneliness, especially if their marriage is full of conflict.[18]

Having different people we can turn to helps us deal with our emotions—a sibling who cheers us up when we're feeling sad, a beloved aunt who calms us when we're feeling anxious, a BFF who grounds us when we're feeling overwhelmed—instead of just relying on one or two people offers a big boost to our well-being.[19]

It also gives our romantic partner, if we have one, a breather from having to absorb all our emotions.

"Friendships give us access to unconditional support as well as practical help in times of stress," says psychologist Linda Sapadin, author of *Now I Get It!: Totally Sensational Advice for Living and Loving.*

"They also expand our lives and let us take on alternate roles apart from coworker, mom or spouse, giving us the chance to grow."[20]

Psychologist Eli J. Finkel calls them Other Significant Others (OSO) in his book *The All-Or-Nothing Marriage*.[21]

Which is exactly what Oprah and Gayle are to each other—they don't look to their romantic and sexual partners to provide all their emotional needs.

All of which points to the need to develop, nurture, and maintain friendships throughout our lives. It's hard to do that if we see women as threats for romantic prospects, as Cindy Gallop expressed in chapter 4. And it doesn't end once a hetero woman has a monogamous partner, philosophy professor Elena Clare Cuffari argues. In her chapter in the anthology *New Philosophies of Sex and Love: Thinking Through Desire*, Cuffari notes that the way society views men is that they need monitoring at all times to make sure they don't "stray." You can probably guess who has the burden of preventing that—their female partner, perpetuating "a culture in which heterosexual women are isolated in suspicion and insecurity." And that inevitably interferes with women's friendships because it sets us up as enemies.[22] Feminists, Cuffari observes, have long noted that "sexism and the zero-sum game for male attention—life under the patriarchy—systematically undermines solidarity and friendship" among women.[23]

Once again, monogamy isn't necessarily a woman's BFF.

It's also hard to nurture female friendships if we're jealous of another woman's wealth, or beauty, or seemingly perfect children and family life, or her accomplishments. Jealousy is among the "Five Friendship Threats," along with judgment, non-reciprocation, neglect, and blame, according to Shasta Nelson, a friendship expert and an author who writes extensively about female friendship.[24]

In truth, research indicates women are much more likely to want to be around other women than men want to be with other men.[25] Many heterosexual women also share more emotional intimacy and have more things in common with their female BFF than their male partner.[26] So with all that going on, what's the problem?

For one, society doesn't give platonic relationships the same kind of acknowledgment, support, or praise as it gives romantic relationships. Just change your *Facebook* status to "in a relationship" or announce your engagement or wedding on Instagram, and the likes, heart emojis, and congratulations will come pouring in. We love a good love story, yet there are amazing but often unspoken stories of how people became friends.

I have one, and it's a story I love to share. As relatively new divorcees at midlife, Kathy and I would meet about once a week at our local coffee shop before we headed off to our respective jobs. One day as we sat there catching up, I sensed the woman sitting at the table next to us, an attractive blonde around our age, was tuning in to our conversation. I immediately felt embarrassed because we were going on and on about men and our latest dating adventures, and it seemed like we were two middle-aged *Sex and the City* divorcée clichés.

Then she leaned over and spoke. Here it comes, I thought.

"Excuse me," she said with a radiant smile. "I'm thinking of moving here and you two look like the kind of women I'd want to know. Can you tell me if this is a good town for single women?"

Kathy and I looked at each other, looked at her, laughed, and said, "Pull up your chair."

That's how we got to know Mary Beth. I like to joke that she picked us up, which is basically what she did. She moved to our town shortly after, and we've been friends ever since.

There's no status update on *Facebook* to announce, "I just met my new BFF," no way to have a friendship that has lasted more than X years be honored, no showers to celebrate making a new friend, or parties to mark the anniversary of a long friendship.

And all of us are worse off because of that.

It puzzles author Andrew Sullivan. "[I]n almost every regard, friendship delivers what love promises but fails to provide," he writes. "Friendship uniquely requires mutual self-knowledge and will. It takes two competent, willing people to be friends. . . . [F]riendship is based on knowledge, and love can be based on mere hope."[27]

When it comes to keeping friendships going, women generally do a better job than men do, especially since the messages we've gotten since childhood from our parents, peers, social institutions, and the mass media emphasize cooperation and emotional support among girls.[28] Women typically are the ones who set the social calendar within heterosexual relationships. Still, there are any number of pressures that threaten those friendships.

All of us are working longer hours at our jobs than ever before, but women also still have what sociologist Arlie Hochschild dubbed "second shifts" at home, although throughout history, many poor and marginalized women have worked multiple shifts that were often invisible and unrecognized.[29] Children (if we have them) demand our time, as do infirm or ill parents, siblings, or other relatives and loved ones who need our care and attention. As do romantic partners. Gen X women, who generally have had children later in life than women in years past, are often juggling all of that at once; they are not called the Sandwich Generation for nothing. Often, women don't even have time for themselves.[30]

Given all that, who can carve out time to call, *FaceTime*, or even text a girlfriend, let alone meet them IRL for coffee, lunch, a gals night, or a getaway? "Every time we get overly busy with work and family, the first thing we do is let go of friendships with other women. We push them right to the back burner," notes Ruthellen Josselson, co-author of *Best Friends: The Pleasures and Perils of Girls' and Women's Friendships.* "That's really a mistake because women are such a source of strength to each other. We nurture one another. And we need to have unpressured space in which we can do the special kind of talk that women do when they're with other women. It's a very healing experience."[31]

The coronavirus pandemic saw many friendships fracture but others strengthen as we shifted our priorities—who do I want to put the time and energy into staying connected to?[32]

And yet, research increasingly indicates there's a need for friends later in life for a host of reasons: well-being, health, caregiving, alleviating social isolation, a buffer against life events that may occur as we age, such as cognitive decline, and even longevity.[33] Hanging with our gal pals also kicks in certain brain chemicals that help us manage the stresses of everyday life—it's more tend and befriend for women than the fight or flight response that appears to be more typical for men.[34]

For women aging without a partner or children, friends aren't relegated to "lesser-than" relationships compared to family or romantic-sexual partnerships—they're seen as being essential to their well-being[35] and for lesbian and bisexual women, the go-to person to count on for informal caregiving.[36] Unfortunately, because society emphasizes the sexual aspect of lesbian relationships—lesbians are defined as "women who have sex with women"—what gets ignored, and thus less supported, is the importance of their female friendships, which reduces those essential relationships to something "less than" the ones they have with women they're sleeping with.[37] But as University of Vermont associate professor Jacqueline S. Weinstock found in her study of midlife lesbians, aged forty to sixty-five, in the United States, there's a strong ethic of friends being family.[38]

University College London professor Roseneil believes the study of female friendship should be the focus of feminist agendas in the twenty-first century, especially since fewer women are marrying and more women are gravitating toward other ways to live, love, and caregive.[39]

All of which means it's time to change the narrative about female friendships at midlife. That's when many women stop seeking approval from others anyway—we're invisible, right?—so midlife is ripe for possibilities to encourage and support each other, to lift each other up, so we can reach our "true potential in terms of aggression, sexuality, and power."

CENTERING FRIENDSHIP

NPR producer and editor Rhaina Cohen presents a case for making friendship, not marriage, the center of our life. Friendships can be as intimate and intertwined as a romantic relationship—all that's missing is sex. Friendship can be "models for how we as a society might expand our conceptions of intimacy and care."[40] As we saw in chapter 3, more and more women will age without children or a romantic partner, and they are looking at various ways to get whatever care they may need.

Philosopher Elizabeth Brake, whom we met in chapter 3 for coining the term "amatonormativity," argues that if the government is going to bestow benefits on people, as it does through marriage, they should go toward supporting caregiving, not a person's romantic or sexual life.[41]

If sex is the big thing privileging romantic relationships over friendships, consider this: many long-term couples stop having sex beginning at midlife—if not earlier. (Just Google "sexless marriage." It's astounding.) So why do we consider the person we have sex with as the most important person in our life? If we stop having sex with that person, but still remain married or in a romantic relationship with them, does that change anything?

And an increasing number of people who identify as asexual or ace, meaning they have little to no sexual attraction to others, or aromantic, meaning they have little to no romantic attraction to others, are marrying their besties as a way to be legally recognized as a family, which gives them access to state and federal perks and privileges, as well as social recognition.[42]

This is why some scholars are suggesting a path toward legally recognizing friendships. One is law professor Laura A. Rosenbury. As she points out, marriage promotes state-supported gendered caregiving while friendship does not. And who typically benefits from that? I'll bet you can guess.

"[I]f individuals want the state to recognize their relationships with other adults, they generally must enter into a marriage or, increasingly, a relationship that mirrors marriage. That encouragement can in turn perpetuate gendered patterns of care because extensive amounts of care are expected of such relationships, and women are still more likely than men to be the primary providers of that care. Friendship, in contrast, does not consistently demand the same amount of care, in part because friendships are not presumed to be exclusive or comprehensive and in part because friendships are presumed to embrace norms of equality and autonomy over norms of domestic dependency."[43]

Rosenbury also notes that women often get more emotional support from their gal pals than they do from their husband or kids. Female friendships also allow them to prioritize the needs of women without feeling obligated to deal with the needs of men or children.[44]

A MIDLIFE LIFELINE

As we've seen, many romantic relationships fall apart starting around midlife. That's when women typically turn back to their female friends for support and intimacy, if they've managed to hold on to them. This is especially true of single mothers, who are often unfairly stigmatized. Reaching out to other single moms can turn that negative perception into a positive, one U.K. study notes. "To a degree, becoming a single mother expanded possibilities and opportunities for intimacies beyond the couple. Moving away from couple relationships—sometimes experienced as insular and limiting—offered an expansion of 'personal communities,' a movement from 'given' (ascribed) ties towards 'chosen' ties based on shared experiences."[45]

I certainly felt that when I divorced at age forty-eight and my boys were still young, nine and twelve. I wasn't exactly a single mother; I was a co-parenting mother. My former husband and I had a fifty-fifty physical custody arrangement; the boys spent a week with him, then a week with me. Still, I was a divorced mother, and there's quite a bit of stigma around divorce (still!) and being a divorcee.

I was not alone, however. I already had a small group of female friends, most of whom I knew since our kids were in kindergarten. Then a few of them divorced around the same time I did, give or take a year or two. Thankfully, most of the ones who were still married didn't abandon us, but you do become a bit of an outsider nonetheless once you become unattached. Couples tend to enjoy doing things with other couples. I understand that, but it's often hurtful and I realized how I had been guilty of that myself when I was married.

At the same time, all my new divorcée friends were eager to find love again, and so our focus wasn't necessarily on strengthening our friendships. It could have slipped back into something more competitive and, in truth, it sometimes did. There were moments of jealousy or sadness when some gals were luckier finding new partners than others.

But then there was a shift when the last of our kids were out of the house for good, and only the adults were left. Each of us had more time, both the empty-nest partnered moms and the empty-nest divorced moms, even though most of us were still working full time. Delightfully, much more of that free time was spent in each other's company. It was if we decided to make our friendships a priority.

There's some science behind that. Midlife is when women start to assess their lives and their friendships, says Suzanna M. Rose, professor of psychology and women's studies at Florida International University, and part of that is often making deliberate and clear-eyed decisions about where to increase and reduce their emotional investment. Old friendships may change or disappear and new ones may arise. But, she notes, the one thing that doesn't change is "the immense importance women attach to their friendships."[46]

The pandemic made it harder for my friends and me to gather like we used to do, of course. So, in the early days of lockdown, we met for hour-long weekly Zoom cocktail hours and sent daily text

threads that kept us laughing, although there also were more se-
rious moments surrounding illnesses, deaths, aging parents. Mostly,
we wanted to stay connected.

As we've slid into our sixties, our conversations more frequently
acknowledge our mortality and imagine our future, individually
and together. Do we create a tiny house community, chip in and
buy a large house or small apartment building, buy houses next to
each other? How do we stay connected to each other and help each
other as we age? Many of us have known each other for two decades
or longer—longer than either of my two marriages. The thought of
moving somewhere with a warmer climate or cheaper living costs
(as tempting as that may sound) where we know no one, as retirees
in my parents' generation often did, is not really how we envision
our future. And if I have to move at some point, I have warned them
that I am taking at least a few of them with me!

We have laughed, cried, comforted, confessed, complained, discussed, celebrated, hiked, vacationed, cooked, and kicked back one
too many glasses of wine together. I would not have been able to
get through my divorce and those hard first few years post-divorce
without them. I can't imagine aging without them.

I want to be near my dear friends, whom I dubbed The Lovelies,
a term that certainly fits each and every one of them. There isn't a
mean girl among them. Not to say that we've always had sunny
times together; it's just that we are willing to embrace the flaws all
of us have and even talk openly about them.

In her 2018 book, *Text Me When You Get Home: The Evolution and
Triumph of Modern Female Friendship,* journalist Kayleen Schaefer
shares that she felt that competition with other girls early on, "for
boys or grades or who looked the prettiest in group pictures."[47]
But as she got older, the competition stopped—women were less a
threat than confidantes, part of a team, a life raft, a soft place to land.

"We're reshaping the idea of what our public support systems
are supposed to look like and what they can be. Women who might
have assumed they could find care, kindness, and deep friendships
are no longer limited to that plotline."[48]

For some that means exploring relationship anarchy, a term
coined by Swedish activist Andie Nordgren whose manifesto promotes the idea that all relationships are equally important, not just
romantic relationships.[49] True, it's outside-the-box thinking, but one
that makes sense as we age because, as psychology lecturer and

sex and gender therapist Meg-John Barker notes, it acknowledges that "platonic relationships can be very important, and that things change over time, so it's important to have freedom and flexibility to keep considering how we manage our relationships."[50]

WHO'S YOUR PERSON?

"'Oh, we're just friends,' is how we talk about our platonic relationships, as if even the closest of our friendships that are not of the exalted romantic variety are not all that valuable. We wonder: Are they relationships of true value?" singles expert and author DePaulo writes in a column asking, "Who's your person," the one you count on to have your back.[51]

Sometimes, "your person" may be a former romantic partner. That's not unusual for lesbian women, who tend to be a lot better in maintaining friendships with former romantic partners than hetero people because creating a sense of community is important for marginalized people.[52]

But, former hetero couples who discover they're better friends than romantic partners can be up to the task, too, and can come together later in life to offer support when it's most needed. That's what happened to Sandra and Daryl Bem, psychology professors whose egalitarian marriage was featured in the inaugural issue of *Ms. Magazine* in 1972, and in her 1998 memoir, *An Unconventional Marriage*.

Even though they had been amicably separated for fifteen years, Daryl took care of Sandra when she was diagnosed with Alzheimer's in 2009. He remained her best friend and one of a handful of close confidantes and helped her end her life as she had wanted to.[53] They did not appear to be having sex.

I admire couples who can do that. While my former husband and I parted relatively amicably, too, and we are friendly—when you have children with someone, you are forever bound—I am not sure we would be able to help each other the same way. And yet more former spouses are showing up as caregivers when one of them becomes gravely ill or is dying. There's a shared intimacy that may be missing from a relationship with a friend.[54]

That said, women tend to expect intimacy in our friendships as we age; we also tend to have higher expectations of our closest friends than men do.[55] We count on our friends for practical things like meals and transportation, advice, and support on everything from relationships to health (who among us hasn't demanded, "Get those chips away from me!" at some point?), and for laughter and conversation. And while many of us prefer to rely on family members for caregiving, calling on friends isn't out of the question.[56] Thankfully, they show up more often than not.

When a friend got breast cancer and, years later, another broke her back in a car accident and then another had knee surgery, The Lovelies jumped into action, making meals, picking up groceries, doing laundry, watering plants, changing sheets. When I broke my left metatarsal and had to wear a boot and use crutches for nine weeks, a Lovely took my dog for long daily walks. We all showed up for each other without having to be asked. Because that's what good friends do.

Studies tell us that divorced and never-married friends tend to give and get more care from each other than married women. Actually, studies say that never-married women do a heck of a lot more caregiving for older adults than women who live with a romantic partner or who are widowed, separated, or divorced.[57]

Can we please give a heartfelt "thank you" to all our single sisters?

That said, in my group of Lovelies, the married women have been as generous with their time and energy in caring for their friends and aging family members as the divorced gals have. I don't think it's just because we're lucky; it's the choice we've made.

YOUNGER, OLDER, DIFFERENT

I almost always start my mornings at the dog park a mile from my house, circling the three-acre expanse a few times so I can get a bit of a workout before I start my workday and my rescue gal Mia can get one, too. There's a senior living home nearby and so many residents stroll around the dog park, which fronts an estuary that attracts all sorts of birds and has magnificent views of my county's tallest peak. I would often see a white-haired, slightly bent over woman walking in the dog park. She always stopped at a certain tree, reaching out her hand and touching it for a few minutes, her head down as if in prayer.

One day, my curiosity got the best of me.

"I hope I'm not being rude, but you always stop at this tree. Is it a special tree?"

"Yes," she told me, her crystal blue eyes almost teary. "This is the tree I would climb if I could."

Well, that nearly busted open my heart. And that's how Jan and I became friends. She was in her mid-eighties at the time.

We'd chat whenever she was at the park and met a few times at a local coffee shop. When the pandemic hit and she couldn't leave the senior living home or have visitors, we emailed each other. I dropped off flowers from time to time; she'd mail me sachets she fashioned using the lavender I gathered from my garden. I got to see the world through her eyes, the world of an older woman that I will be one day—if I'm lucky enough to live to my eighties.

Laura is another friend I've gotten to know at the dog park (if you want to make friends, get a dog—really). Laura is in her early seventies, a few years older than I am, and a lesbian. Our conversations have been varied, intimate, enlightening, and entertaining.

These women, these accidental friendships, have greatly enriched me. Having friends of different ages and life experiences will do that. If only those kinds of friendships were encouraged and supported.

My friendship with Inka—a big, beautiful, German-born single mom who just turned forty—developed organically, too. She's been cutting and highlighting my hair for years, but we might as well be each other's shrinks given how deep and intimate our conversations have gotten over the years. Almost all her friendships are with older women because she learns from them and there isn't as much BS, she tells me. I've met some at the weekly Thursday happy hours she hosted on her apartment complex's front lawn last spring and summer.

Inka's among just a handful of friendships I have with women younger than I am, although I am close with some of my friends' daughters, now in their late twenties and early thirties, who went to school with my boys.

It's been harder to meet younger women who don't have some sort of connection with me, whether through my kids or work. That said, I suppose I could get as creative as journalist Rachel Bertsche has been.

Bertsche had a unique idea. When she moved with her soon-to-be husband to Chicago, where she knew no one, she was desperate to meet women she could call friends. So, she reached out to her social network asking for the names of women they knew who lived in the area, and humorously describes her search in her 2012 book, *MWF Seeking BFF: My Yearlong Search for a New Best Friend*. She set up lunch dates with several women, including a forty-something single mom of two tweens. But Bertsche's coworkers teased her for attempting to make friends with a woman more than a decade older than she is. Bertsche met her anyway, had a dinner or two after, but relatively quickly dismissed her. She foresaw a worrisome future that most likely included having to attend high school volleyball games and dance recitals.

"What kind of a friendship is really possible with a mom of puberty-crazed children? I'm almost embarrassed—how are we going to look, me and the mom?" she writes. "I'm not exactly sure why I'm hung up on the age and kids thing. Maybe I'm trying to hold onto my youth. Like being best friends with a woman about 13 years closer to middle age would make *me* seem closer to middle age. . . . While friends with babies seems doable, friends with teenagers seems, well, old."[58]

What a missed opportunity! If she's lucky, Bertsche will one day be a middle-aged woman herself, perhaps with a puberty-crazed kid or two, and perhaps even a middle-aged single mom due to divorce or death. There are no givens in life except, as we are told, death and taxes. Would that forty-something middle-aged single mom be a role model or even a peek into some future self Bertsche may or may not be? Could be. We'll never know. Bertsche may have viewed her potential older friend as a woman who would need something from her (baby-sitting perhaps, or someone to sit next to her on the volleyball court bleachers) instead of thinking of her as someone who can offer help, thereby ignoring and missing out on the potential for mutual support.[59]

Younger women may diss older women, but that works at all ages, as Jeannie Ralston, editor and co-founder of NextTribe.com, a digital magazine for women over forty-five, discovered. In her desire to befriend the younger women in her Zumba class, only to be dismissed by them, she realizes she had been "guilty of the very sin I felt had been committed against me. I was overlooking the other women, especially those older than me—women in their late 60s, 70s or even 80s."

Why did she do that? "Maybe subconsciously we still want to be in the cool group like in high school. We want to surround ourselves with people who reflect well on us."[60]

Does hanging around with younger women reflect well on their older sisters? Do they make us feel or seem more youthful? Are all young women "cool"? Are all women in their sixties, seventies, and eighties uncool? I have questions!

In many other countries, multigenerational living brings young and old together. That isn't as common in the United States but it has been growing in recent years, although often more out of necessity than desire.[61] Perhaps that's why there's been a rise in intergenerational women's groups and gatherings, at least until the pandemic hit. As the founder of one such gathering notes, bringing women of different ages together helps younger women understand that "one day they will be older women and that we're all responsible for creating a society that honors older women."[62]

We are indeed responsible for creating that society, not only for ourselves but also for all women. We will spend many of our later years in each other's company, after all.

Intergenerational friendships offer big perks for both older and younger women, according to an AARP study. Both can benefit by seeing things from a different perspective, as I have with Jan, until she died in the fall of 2021, and Laura. Older friends can inspire younger women and act as role models, whereas having younger friends offers older women a chance to share the wisdom of their years. Perhaps most importantly, intergenerational friendships could go a long way toward busting ageist beliefs, and even offer younger women a more positive attitude about aging, which is what we want, right?[63]

And it works in reverse. One study of Black women in their sixties and older indicates that having more positive expectations about growing older made it easier for them to make new friends and feel like they could count on them for support.[64] It seems like a win-win.

"Bridging the generation gap not only increases the friend pool, but it also expands and supports mental well-being," says Anna Kudak, coauthor of *What Happy Women Do*. "Friendships with older and younger people help broaden your perspective, which in turn allows you to have compassion and empathy in your day-to-day life."[65]

That said, most of us tend to make friends with women who are like us, not only in age, but also in race and class. They're often the people we meet in our religious and civic activities, in our neighborhoods or local eateries or coffee shops, or at work. If those are not places rich in diversity, that may limit our chances of meeting women whose experiences of aging might be different than our own.

Kersha Smith, who is Black, and Marcella Runell Hall, who is White, bonded over first-time motherhood many years ago although the two academics knew many of the same people and even lived around the corner from each other. Now in their mid-forties, their friendship has endured. That isn't all that typical, as they discovered while gathering narratives for the book they co-edited, *UnCommon Bonds: Women Reflect on Race and Friendship*. Among the topics they wanted to address in their book was why women's friendships "become more narrow and homogenous" as they age.[66]

Because they do, although narrowing doesn't always mean it's a negative thing. It's true that our social networks decline as we age, but often it's because we ditch the friends who are draining—and you know *exactly* who they are—and spend more time with the women who are our closest and most emotionally rewarding friends. However, our friendships also narrow because of things out of our control—death, illness, retirement, a move, or diminished financial resources, which might limit our ability to get together for a coffee, hike, or gals getaway.[67]

Our friendships become homogenous for a variety of reasons, racial bias among them, although often we just don't live near or work with one another. There may be a lack of trust or a disconnect, as two women in *UnCommon Bonds* share in their essay.[68] And it often isn't promoted. "This country has a pretty long history of restriction on inter-racial contact and for Whites and Blacks, even though it's in the past, there are still echoes of this," sociologist Ann Morning tells the *Reuters* news agency.[69] And we are the poorer for that.

Women typically have fewer friends of another race at midlife than men have, although Asian, Latina, and multiracial women tend to have more diverse friends than either White or Black women. The reasons are varied and complex, but trust has a lot to do with it. Still, whatever cross-racial friends we do have tend to be deeper, more intimate friendships.[70]

Expanding on what author Kudak says, having diverse friends as we age would go far toward helping us be compassionate toward each other (and ourselves), and expand our beliefs about aging and what it's "supposed" to be like, especially since it's projected that by 2044, non-Hispanic White people will be a minority in the United States.[71]

The older we get, the more marginalized we become in this society, even women who may not have been marginalized before.
Having diverse female friends would help us be better allies in the
fight against ageism, racism, sexism, and all the other "isms" we'd
like to dismantle and make for a more inclusive society.

I'M FINE ON MY OWN

After all my chatting up the importance of female friendships, here
comes the big downer: Not every woman needs or wants them.
A twenty-year study of older people in rural Wales found that although they were physically isolated, they didn't feel lonely. They
enjoyed their own company, thank you very much.[72] Granted, that
feeling may be unique to Wales, a country whose people have been
called by *The Guardian*—not me!—"temperamental."[73] Still, many
women are good at being their own source of comfort and security.[74]
They may not need or want a lot of friends, and they may prefer
male friends over female friends, especially as they age.

"It's emotionally exhausting to try to make new connections,
especially when you're content with the ones you already have,"
says Laura L. Carstensen, a professor of psychology at Stanford
University and director of its Center on Longevity. "We live in a
more-is-better culture. We're generally brought up to believe that if
a little bit of something is good, then a lot of it must be better. But
that's not necessarily true when it comes to friends."[75]

And female friendships can sometimes become—and I am saying
this as kindly as I can—complicated. As mentioned above, women
have high expectations of their female friends.[76] We're more likely
to attribute whatever friendship problems we have to—ahem—our
friends' character quirks, not anything about us. And, somewhat
surprisingly, sometimes the more friends older women have, the
more problems they're likely to have with them.[77]

There isn't much research on the darker sides of friendship later
in life—you know, the friends who give us more grief than pleasure
but we're loath to break up with anyway. Let's face it—there isn't
much research on later-life friendships, period, despite its importance for a rapidly growing aging population.[78] Again, it points
out how older people are ignored and dismissed—call it what it is,
ageism.

But one thing seems to be consistent. Rather than confront our friends when we feel like they've hurt or disappointed us, no matter how openly and lovingly we can do that, many older women still choose to say nothing so we can avoid conflict with the women we've called friends.[79] Which once again speaks to the need to openly talk about our disagreements, disappointments, and anger in healthy ways so we can bust that narrative of being mean girls. Channeling *The Golden Girls* Dorothy and Blanche might help. Not Mean Girls, but Golden Girls.

I have gotten better at this with my gal friends. I love them all, yet after being friends for decades I know which ones I can ask for or share honest observations, secrets, and other intimate conversations. I have been delightfully surprised by how that has shape shifted with some, because I'd never experienced them that way before. I always try to be that friend, but I am sure I have failed at times— OK, many times. Good friends seem to accept each other even when they are aware of each other's faults and shortcomings. The bigger picture—*do I truly value this woman and want her in my life*—is what matters.

Regardless of the narratives and the research, you are the best person to ask about what you want, and don't want, from your female friends as you age; how many friendships you can reasonably maintain, based on your time and energy; and how many friends you truly want to be close to; whether you are available to show up for them for informal caregiving and whether you'd feel comfortable asking for help, or receiving help, from them. In other words, how willing are you to explore what friendship means to you and how that might change as you age?

THINGS TO THINK ABOUT

What role has friendship played in your life?
Which friend is your closest confidante and why?
Has it been easy or hard to make new friends or keep the ones you have? Why?
Do you feel comfortable asking for, or receiving help from friends?
How do you see your need for friendship changing as you age?

6

✛

"It's Probably Just Your Hormones"

Certainly the effort to remain unchanged, young, when the body gives so impressive a signal of change as the menopause, is gallant; but it is a stupid, self-sacrificial gallantry, better befitting a boy of twenty than a woman of forty-five or fifty. Let the athletes die young and laurel-crowned. Let the soldiers earn the Purple Hearts. Let women die old, white-crowned, with human hearts.

—Ursula K. Le Guin, author[1]

In her street clothes, she looked like the quintessential "little old lady," a diminutive, seemingly frail older woman with likely not much to offer.

"Her appearance allowed people to make her into an affectionate doll. . . . She was made cute and sweet and accessible," is how journalist Janice Kaplan describes her.[2]

The "little old lady" was the late Supreme Court Justice Ruth Bader Ginsburg, who died in 2020 at age eighty-seven.

A relentless advocate for women's rights and social issues with a whip-smart brain, the Notorious RBG, as she was known, was a force to be reckoned with, but she didn't look like it, even when she was appointed to the high court at age sixty. It would be all too easy to write her off as someone's doddering but beloved Bubbie by her appearance alone, especially wearing her lacy jabots, gloves, scrunchies, and eyeglasses.

How wrong they'd be!

And yet older women who look just like RBG are often viewed in the worst possible way. In addition to wrinkles, skin spots, gray hair, and all the other visible signs of aging, older people in general are seen as forgetful, passive, weak, feeble, frail, debilitated, disabled, dependent, and depressed. Seen through the lens of sexism that women have long had to deal with—the ideal feminine woman is considered naturally weak, frail, passive, and dependent—it's no wonder that as women age, we're more often thought to be incompetent and deserving of pity than older men are.

In fact, viewing "little old ladies" as kind, sweet, nurturing, and helpful is a form of benevolent ageism, the kind of ageism that seems like people are being gracious, but are actually patronizing us in a way that can have negative physical and mental health consequences.[3] It also sets up women to internalize "the best justification for gender inequality: incompetence."[4]

As a fighter for gender equality, RBG clearly did not show any signs of incompetence. Still, not all older women have her strength, support, and sheer chutzpah to counteract the messaging.

Like all the other disturbing narratives we've covered in this book so far, women's perceived frailty has real-life consequences on our health and our experiences in the health-care system. (For the record, just 7 percent of women older than sixty-five, not living in nursing homes or hospitals, are actually considered frail.[5])

According to a study led by Joan C. Chrisler, founding editor of the journal *Women's Reproductive Health*—pointedly named "Ageism Can Be Hazardous to Women's Health: Ageism, Sexism, and Stereotypes of Older Women in the Healthcare System"—internalized ageist and negative stereotypes can become self-fulfilling prophecies for women, often leading us to learned helplessness and perceived bad health.[6] So if we think we might not be able to do certain things, say follow complicated medication directions or navigate an iPhone upgrade, then we're actually more likely to not be able to do them. A self-fulfilling prophecy indeed. And since there's a long history of doctors and other health-care specialists being dismissive of women's pain and discomfort, and often misdiagnosing our medical issues such as heart attacks, this is worrisome, especially since we live longer than men do and thus have many more years dealing with the health-care system as "old" people.[7]

This is not to say that some women don't become weak, frail, and dependent as they age. Of course they do. Many also develop one or more disabilities, as we saw earlier in the book, as well as cognitive issues, and bone and heart diseases as well as a host of other ailments.

It's just that in addition to internalizing the damaging stereotypes about older women and dealing with a dismissive health-care system, women also often struggle hard for years—and spend a crapload of money—trying not to look their age.

Add all those things together and the impacts on us are much more than skin deep.

"Age denial keeps many people from making lifestyle choices that pay off in the long run," writes anti-ageism activist Ashton Applewhite.[8] Think about it: What helpful and harmful lifestyle decisions are women making or avoiding in their effort to remain looking young?

It's totally understandable that women are often into age denial. After all, there's a huge pressure for us to do whatever we can to remain or become beautiful, stay fit and youthful looking, and we're judged much more harshly than men are once we start to show even the tiniest hint of aging.[9]

What does that mean? All that judgment takes a toll on us. As Chrisler and her team note, "older women who are subjected to greater age discrimination may experience poorer health and lower body esteem. Consequently, women's psychological well-being may be negatively affected by both ageist discrimination and low body esteem."[10]

I'm sure I'm not the only older woman who doesn't feel my age. I look it, sure; I have the wrinkles, the sagging, the age spots, and in the what-fresh-hell-is-this category, the jowls, to prove I'm a sixty-something woman. But inside, I still feel a lot like my younger, spunky, former hippie self; I'm just not wearing tie-dye, hip-huggers, and love beads anymore, which is a very good thing. According to studies, feeling younger than our actual age, our so-called subjective age, offers mental and physical health perks. Clearly, there's something to the cliché that you're only as old as you feel.[11]

If we enter midlife feeling pretty good about ourselves, it actually positively impacts our health—things like cardiovascular issues, memory, balance, hospitalizations, and even the will to live and mortality—as many as forty years later. And if we're optimistic about our future selves, aging doesn't seem all that bad. But there's one thing that gets in our way: internalized ageist stereotypes. Even joking about our "senior moments" of forgetfulness—and who doesn't do that?—hurts us because it reinforces the idea that having a bad memory is something a woman our age is destined to have.[12]

Ageist discrimination leads to stress, and stress is really bad for our health; it negatively impacts our immune system and can be a contributing factor to developing some chronic illnesses or worsen ones we already have.[13]

By midlife, Black women are biologically seven and a half years "older" than White women, due in great part to perceived stress as well as poverty, research indicates.[14] A lifetime of exposure to systemic racism also leads to physical stress, metabolic dysfunction, and mental health challenges for Black women.[15]

If ageism hits us after a lifetime of other types of discrimination we've been subjected to, from sexism to racism to homophobia to ableism to transphobia to fatphobia—and some women experience several types of discrimination at the same time due to the intersectionality of their identities—is it any wonder that our physical and mental health may suffer?[16]

If society really believes older women are weak, frail, passive, and dependent, well, forcing us to deal with all that judgment is a surefire way to actually make us weak, frail, passive, and dependent. Mission accomplished! Nice going, guys.

What if we got different messages? What if we didn't feel so pressured to deny our age and feel shame about our womanhood? What if we had a health-care system that was interested in understanding and knowledgeable about caring for women's bodies and minds, and actually listened to us? What kind of decisions would we make to feel healthy as we age?

Ageism hits women early. *Facebook* chief executive officer Sheryl Sandberg admitted in 2021 that she was considered "middle-aged" at the social media giant, and by extension all of Silicon Valley and young male-heavy tech companies everywhere, when she hit thirty-five—thirty-five![17] Now that she's in her early fifties, she actually *is* squarely in middle age and no doubt in the throes of menopause. And if there's any time when a woman's health comes into play (assuming she doesn't enter midlife already having health issues or disabilities or both) it's menopause.

MENOPAUSAL MAYHEM

Menopause is having a hot moment of late. There have been dozens of articles in the past few years with headlines announcing "Why Everyone Needs to Know More About Menopause—Especially Now" *(Washington Post)*, "Why Modern Medicine Keeps Overlooking Menopause" *(New York Times)*, "Menopause is Having a Moment" *(Vox)*, and "Of Course Gen X Is Doing Menopause Differently" *(InStyle)*, as well as a spate of new books.

It may be because Gen X women, who are just now hitting midlife and well on their way to perimenopause and menopause—the average age of menopause in the United States is fifty-one—grew up using social media and are amplifying their voices on various platforms with a collective, "What the hell is going on with me?"

Whatever the reason, thank goodness it's happening because up until recently, there's been a dearth of open, honest, and accurate conversation about this very natural phase of a woman's life.

Oh, we hear plenty about menopausal symptoms—the hot flashes, the sleepless nights, the moods, the weight gain, the sweating, brain fog, vaginal dryness, yada, yada, yada. And not every woman experiences all of those symptoms, and some women may have mild symptoms, or some mild and some severe—it's highly individual. What we don't hear nearly enough, if at all, is how menopause impacts a woman's health.

In a word, huge.

As Dr. Jen Gunter, a San Francisco Bay Area OB-GYN, writes, while a woman's last period is generally what's considered the pièce de résistance of menopause, it is hardly the main event. "[W]hat really matters for the day-to-day lives of people with ovaries starts years before the final menstrual period and lasts a lifetime, as the hormonal changes of the transition can increase women's risk of conditions such as heart disease, stroke, dementia and osteoporosis," and could shorten her lifespan or negatively affect her quality of life.[18]

I had no knowledge of the health risks outside of osteoporosis when I started menopause, even though I had a savvy gynecologist. Zip. Nada.

Sadly, I was not alone in that.

"Until internists and family medicine doctors see menopause as a threat to health in general, they're not going to take it seriously."

They're going to say, "This is one of those female things that will go away. That's contributed to this gap in knowledge in terms of physicians and other practitioners and this 'menopause management vacuum,'" says Dr. Stephanie S. Faubion, director of the Mayo Clinic's Center for Women's Health and medical director for the North American Menopause Society.[19]

What kind of gap in knowledge? According to Faubion, a 2018 survey of family medicine, internal medicine, and obstetrics and gynecology residency trainees say they had about one or two total hours of education about menopause, max, and some 20 percent said they'd had no menopause education at all. None! This is one of the most major health events in a woman's life, and it's very likely her health-care provider knows little to nothing about it, and how to best help her.

This does not inspire much confidence.

And that's just for cis hetero women. There's even less knowledge for queer people, even though those entering midlife now include a much larger percentage of non-binary people, trans women on hormone replacement therapy, and trans men than in any previous generation. For Black and Latina women, who start menopause two years earlier than White women do, according to research, and also experience more severe symptoms such as hot flashes and night sweats (along with Native American women), the need for savvy health-care providers matters a lot.[20] Same for the growing number of childless and childfree women, because research shows that women who have never given birth or been pregnant have twice the chance of starting menopause before they hit age forty, putting them at a higher risk of heart attacks, strokes, osteoporosis, and type 2 diabetes.[21] Disabled women also hit menopause earlier, around age fifty, which can accelerate bone loss.[22]

If our health-care providers are often at a loss to guide us, imagine our poor male romantic/sexual partners (if we have them). Actually, imagine poor us having to live with someone who has little to no idea about what's going on with us and what to expect during menopause. That could interfere with our sexual desire and pleasure.

If women struggle with understanding menopause, how can we expect our male partners (if we're hetero) to support us—or at least not get frustrated with us, which just further complicates an already often confusing and taboo process that is still considered a big bummer.

And it is a big bummer for many women. There's a lot of shame, stigma, and misunderstanding around menopause, just as it is around menstruation, and that impacts what we think and how we act. When we were younger, we worried about leaking when we got our period. At midlife, we worry about having a hot flash during an important presentation at work, or at a parent-teacher conference, or on a date, leading us women to be hyper-vigilant, self-conscious, and self-monitoring. It's exhausting.[23] No surprise, then, that women who have a sour attitude toward menopause overwhelmingly have more problematic menopausal symptoms.[24]

That sets off a whole chain of relationship challenges and furthers the stereotypes about middle-aged women.

According to one study, more men whose partners were experiencing some of the symptoms of menopause said they were more negatively impacted by the symptoms than their partners were—an interesting factoid for sure. More than half also said it was putting a strain on their relationship. Thankfully, most men (correctly) attributed their partner's symptoms to menopause, but disturbingly about 22 percent attributed the symptoms to aging, or menopause *and* aging. Aging? If a guy isn't experiencing hot flashes, night sweats, and moodiness at midlife, why the heck would he think that's how aging impacts a woman? And if he does think that, how might that influence how he views other women, say his female coworkers or a potential female hire? That could be very, very problematic for the women.[25]

And the moodiness bothers them; in fact, the same study found that if men were going to explain to another guy what menopause is all about, some 22 percent would say it causes a lot of moodiness and irrational behavior.

But they were trying to be more patient, supportive, and compassionate toward their partner, or at least a third of them said so; 11 percent said were just trying to avoid the whole thing.[26]

Perhaps that's why early types of hormone replacement therapy to alleviate menopausal symptoms were typically marketed not to women, but to their husbands, according to British scholar Elinor Cleghorn.[27]

Clearly, men need help understanding menopause beyond just their female partner's symptoms. But maybe they should also be a tad more concerned about how it may impact her health. I guarantee you that poor health will have a *much* bigger impact on their relationship.

If our male romantic partner is clueless about that and our health-care provider isn't talking about that with us or is just chalking it up to "one of those female things that will go away," and if we ourselves are hesitant to ask about it—and who wouldn't be if our doctor is being so dismissive?—we will truly continue to perpetuate the dangerous ageist narratives about us and thus the health of our older selves is going to be severely disadvantaged.

No thanks.

Throughout history, the stories women share about their experiences with the health-care system have a common thread: "women not being listened to, women being misdiagnosed, women being in pain and being told that they were anxious or stressed," Cleghorn says.[28]

She knows that firsthand.

PATHOLOGIZING "FEMALENESS"

When Cleghorn started getting leg pains and swelling in her ankle in her twenties, her male doctor first suggested it might be gout. Or was she perhaps pregnant? "I can see nothing wrong with you. It's probably just your hormones," he tells her.

It wasn't her hormones, it was systemic lupus erythematosus, which wasn't diagnosed until, at age thirty, she had suffered nearly a decade of pain, a story she details in her book *Unwell Women: Misdiagnosis and Myth in a Man-Made World.*[29] As she notes, about 4 percent of people around the world suffer from an autoimmune disease like hers, and 80 percent are women.[30]

While we no longer blame woman's ills on her uterus—with marriage and motherhood believed to be the cure to a misbehaving womb—our hormones now seem to be the troublemakers. Or our weight. Or our age. Or our overactive mind. "Medicine has insisted on pathologizing 'femaleness,' and by extension womanhood," Cleghorn writes.[31]

Imagine how much physical pain and mental distress women have gone through in years past and continue to go through because of that belief.

"We have moved on exponentially over the centuries in our attitudes toward gender and our understanding what a human body is, but because those attitudes are so ingrained, they've shaped a lot of the understanding of diseases from a clinical perspective" she says. "Statistically, it's been shown that if a woman presents with chronic pain that doesn't have an immediately diagnostic cause, she's more likely to be seen as having a mental health condition than to be referred for further tests. She's much more likely to be dismissed with a recommendation of a sedative or an antidepressant medicine than an analgesic or opioid pain medication, which men would be offered."[32]

In her study on ageism, Chrisler also found that the belief that older women are frail could actually prevent a health-care provider from recommending an aggressive treatment such as joint replacement surgery even though women are much more likely to have knee and hip arthritis and other types of joint issues, or heart bypass surgery and other heart therapies even when their conditions are similar to a man's.[33]

So, are older women truly weak, frail, passive, incompetent, and dependent, or are we being seen by society and treated that way by the health-care providers we rely on? Could it be that the perceptions of menopausal women—our moodiness, depression, and being perpetually pissed off—and the perceived frailty of older women might have something to do with us feeling unheard, dismissed, and patronized by the very people we turn to for help?

"If the stereotype is to think women are more expressive than men, perhaps 'overly' expressive, then the tendency will be to discount women's pain behaviors," says Elizabeth Losin, director of the Social and Cultural Neuroscience lab at the University of Miami, whose research found that when men and women complained about the same amount of pain, the women's pain was believed to be less intense than the men's. The suggested treatment? Psychotherapy, not medication, meaning it's probably all in her head.[34]

I would complain that all of this is giving me a royal pain in the neck, but I fear no one will believe me.

Of course, it isn't just our pain that's discounted. Because the narrative about older women is that we lose interest in sex and thus aren't seen as sexual beings even though many of us are happily getting it on, as we saw in chapter 2, there's a huge rise in sexually transmitted infection (STIs) lately. In fact, STIs have more than doubled in the past decade in the United States among adults age sixty-five years and older, especially among widows and divorcees.[35]

There has been a spate of news stories in recent years about the rise of sexually transmitted diseases in nursing homes and care facilities, again because of ageist beliefs that older people aren't doing it. Except they are.[36]

Women are at a particularly higher risk because the tissues of the vagina and vulva get thinner and drier after menopause, which can lead to micro-abrasions, creating a welcoming environment for an infection. Some medications can further thin the tissues.[37]

Part of the problem is that few are aware of the risks of contracting an STI, what it looks like, what the symptoms are, how it's transmitted, and how it's treated.[38] The other part of the problem is that Medicare only mandates a doctor to assess an older person's vision, hearing, memory, and balance. There's no such requirement to ask a patient about her sex life. So, if a doctor thinks their female patient is asexual because she's "old," and she doesn't ask because she might feel awkward—or shamed—for asking about sex, she could end up in trouble.

Again, the narratives about aging as a woman can hurt us, and when they relate to our health, possibly kill us.

THE PROBLEM WITH AGING SUCCESSFULLY

I'm now in my mid-sixties and here's what's happened in the past decade or so. I went from 1.0 drugstore reading glasses to progressively stronger prescription reading glasses as well as prescription distance glasses. My night vision has gotten so bad that I basically had to stop driving past sunset and hopefully by now have had cataract surgery. I walk at least an hour a day—that's what having a dog will do—as well as bicycle at least once a week, lift weights, and eat a healthy, low-carb, mostly plant-based diet, and yet I still put on about ten pounds that have given me that familiar thick midlife female stomach (although on the plus side, my bra size went from an A to B cup; I finally have cleavage). I've shrunk almost a full inch from my former tallish five-foot-eight-inch physique. That pain in my neck that I thought was just from sitting for hours in front of my computer? It's actually arthritis. Oh hello, chronic pain.

I was a typical woman at midlife, when disabilities start to kick in.[39]

I had to wonder: Was I aging successfully?

When I first heard the term, I thought it meant staying as healthy as you can for as long as you can, which made a lot of sense to me. I was trying to. I sure didn't plan to have crappy eyesight but that's genetics—hey, thanks Mom—or become arthritic, but I'm not sure I had any say in that. But I was wrong about what aging successfully is.

The concept dates back to the 1960s, when Robert J. Havighurst, an expert on human development and aging, posited that aging can be a positive thing. But it really took off in 1998 with the publication of *Successful Aging,* by Dr. John W. Rowe and psychologist Robert L. Kahn, based on the results of the MacArthur Foundation Study of Aging in America. Their take on aging successfully came with a few mandates—avoiding disease and disability at all cost, staying mentally and physically fit, engaging in all life has to offer, and being a productive member of society. We see this play out in ads, with happy older people—mostly White hetero couples, because that's the heteronormative idealized norm—jogging, caring for grandkids, dancing, hiking, and holding hands while walking on the beach, a particularly popular image. They may not be young anymore, but they sure are active and youthful! And, they have a romantic partner, of course. Can a single woman *really* be happy later in life?

On the surface aging successfully sounds great, but what happens if you happen to become disabled, or are born with a disability? What if you were never physically fit, perhaps because of health issues, and so may be unlikely to suddenly become fit at midlife? What if you want to be productive but caregiving responsibilities prevent you from remaining in the workplace or volunteering? Do you have any hope of aging well?

The worst part of their concept of successful aging is that the good doctors put it all in our hands. It's our fault if we don't age well, as if government policies and the various inequities that created ageism in the first place have absolutely nothing to do with our actual experience of aging.[40] Now who's wrong?

Which is why it's wise not to mention "successful aging" to Martha Holstein.

"We don't have successful middle age. We don't have successful childhood," observes Holstein, one of America's foremost scholars on feminist gerontology. "Successful aging is a concept that says there's a bad way to age, and there's a good way to age. So I don't want any adjective except to recognize that being old is as diverse and as interesting or boring as any age."[41]

If my crappy eyesight, lethargic metabolism, and arthritic neck mean I'm somehow failing at aging successfully, I would like to talk to the manager.

While the concept of aging successfully impacts both men and women with its classist, ableist, and, let's admit it, downright shaming messaging, it impacts women more—of course!—because it perpetuates gender stereotypes that emphasize beauty and youth, both of which are impossible to hold on to.

As we explored in chapter 4, women feel a lot of pressure to be beautiful and stay fit for as long as possible in order to look anything but their age, often at great financial, physical, and emotional cost. It's a lifelong project that takes more and more work as we age. While some women at midlife experience a shift in how they think about their bodies, focusing a little less on what it looks like and a little more on the fact that they have a body that works, thank goodness, they come up against a culture that doesn't place the same kind of value on a functioning body over a youthful one.[42]

Look, we're not dummies. Older women are acutely aware of how our body "should" look, so it's understandable why some of us may begin (or continue) to feel bad about our body. And that leads to depression and other types of psychological distress.[43]

Aging successfully still is all about sexualizing a woman's body.

"The question of how successfully a woman conforms to traditional, heterosexual norms of femininity—is she physically attractive? sexually desirable? reproductively viable?—remains an influential measure, albeit not the only measure, of a woman's individual and social value in contemporary American culture," writes Abigail T. Brooks, director of the Women's Studies Program and assistant professor of sociology at Providence College.[44]

How can a woman age successfully if she looks her age, no matter how healthy she is? She can't. It seems that women are aged more by cultural narratives than by aging itself.[45]

And if you're not a cis hetero White woman, aging successfully takes on different meanings.

We already saw how the Strong Black Woman stereotype can hurt Black women economically, but it can also impact their health in ways both positive and negative. Being a Strong Black Woman means you're strong, independent, resilient, and able to handle any challenge, whether psychological or physical. Internalizing that narrative can take a psychological and physical toll on Black women, studies have found. At the same time, the belief in one's independence, strength, and resilience can give a Black woman a sense of mastery over her life and confidence to overcome obstacles that can help her age as best she can.[46]

It's similar for the estimated 2.4 million lesbian and bisexual women in the United States aged fifty and older. The impacts of living outside the heterosexual norm are stressful, and that puts them at a greater risk of physical disabilities, poor mental health, obesity, and cardiovascular disease than hetero women, which would seem to exclude them from the rules of successful aging. And yet a study of older lesbian and bisexual women found that many experience the same resilience Black women have. As the study's lead author, Jennifer M. Jabson Tree, an associate professor at the University of Tennessee in Knoxville observes, older sexual minority women (SMW) "have existed for many years in a culture that is unfriendly and unaccepting to their identity, their values, and their life choices. This might be translated into better ways of coping for SMW with the decrements that aging brings, even optimal aging."[47]

If successful aging truly means avoiding a disability, well, what if you're already disabled? While new technologies aimed at aging able-bodied Boomers in recent years have benefited disabled people, too, they've done little to dismantle the harmful stereotypes disabled older women have had to deal with.

Women with physical or cognitive disabilities are more than twice as likely as able-bodied women to experience health challenges that could put them at a greater risk of cardiovascular disease.[48] A study by the Center for Research on Women with Disabilities found that many women with physical disabilities also live with chronic urinary tract infections, heart disease, depression, and osteoporosis at younger ages than able-bodied women. Some were even refused care by a physician because of the type of disability they had.[49]

Still, the late Margaret A. Nosek, the center's founder and executive director, was hopeful. In that study, Nosek and her team found that women with disabilities were "triumphant" over negative stereotypes. Asexual? Dependent? Nope. How about resilient?

Seventy-eight percent of the women surveyed said they had high or moderately high self-esteem.

It's interesting that the women who have been most marginalized by society have found an inner strength and flexibility to feel good in their own skin.

"People like me, born disabled, with progressively more health conditions, were never supposed to live this long, but we are. Contrary to expectations and stereotypes, we are living well and maintaining our productivity as long as we are connected with state-of-the-art medicine and technology," Nosek wrote in 2006, when she was fifty-four, fourteen years before her death.[50]

Gen Xers, she notes, grew up expecting ramps, curb cuts, and handicapped parking. Millennials are driving a queer crip fashion movement that's disrupting cultural norms around the body and identity and making fashion accessible to all.[51] "A cane, a wheelchair, or even a ventilator no longer needs to symbolize decline or end of life. Somewhere in the last half-century, we learned to define ourselves beyond the expectations of others, reject stereotypes, and not be afraid to demand answers."

That's a great message for all women at midlife and older, abled and disabled. We live longer than men do and thus are more likely to develop one or more disabilities later in life. We will have many years to deal with a society and health-care system that has often been dismissive of us and, according to Nosek, is not ready to care for the inevitable rise in the number of women with disabilities in the coming decades. One thing her study couldn't predict is the coronavirus pandemic and the lingering effects on those who contract COVID-19, the so-called long haulers. Recent studies indicate that women are much more likely to be long haulers than men are, often impacting their ability to work.[52] We just don't know what that means for the future.

In order to "define ourselves beyond the expectations of others, reject stereotypes, and not be afraid to demand answers," we'll need to push past our own prejudices about disability first. We have work to do.

Remember—by 2030 there will be more women in the United States between the ages of forty and sixty-four than girls under the age of eighteen, according to Census Bureau projections.[53] We may not want to "age successfully" as that's currently defined, but how about aging as best we can on our own terms?

"I'm not afraid of dying," writes Jennifer Burgmann, who became disabled at age thirty-eight and whom we met in chapter 4. "I'm afraid of not living well."[54]

Me, too.

THINGS TO THINK ABOUT

What are your biggest health concerns about aging?

What are your biggest concerns about menopause?

What stereotypes do you have about how women age physically and mentally?

In what ways has aging impacted your mental and physical health?

In what ways do you feel prepared or not for your future physical and mental self?

7

✝

Investments Are
a Girl's Best Friend

I truly believe that women should be financially independent from their men. And let's face it, money gives men the power to run the show. It gives men the power to define value. They define what's sexy. And men define what's feminine.

—Beyoncé, singer-songwriter[1]

The year I turned nineteen, I dropped out of the University of Vermont and followed my boyfriend to Colorado, where he was going to attend the Colorado School of Mines. I didn't know that I was going to end up supporting him, as well as our two dogs, cat, and snake, with my minimum-wage jobs because his parents—churchgoing Catholics—were not hip to couples living together unless they were married. But I didn't care; we were two young idealistic and in love hippies who spent our weekends hiking in the Rockies with our pups. We eventually did get married, just a few months shy of my twenty-first birthday, but somehow I still ended up supporting him while he basically attended P.E. classes.

We were poor, but money didn't really matter all that much to me then. We had enough to get by, and life felt rich in so many other ways.

Still, all those years of working minimum-wage jobs were a drag. And, at the same time, an eye-opening experience—one I hope to never have to repeat. Yet it's where women often find themselves.

Women overwhelmingly work low-paying jobs—child and elder care workers, restaurant servers, maids, teachers, cashiers, retail workers, receptionists—and as little as those jobs pay, Black woman, women of color, and women with disabilities make even less than White women. Same with even better-paying careers. Only lesbians seem to fare well compared with their hetero sisters, but still, of course, not better than men, straight or gay.[2]

How did women get to this place?

You most likely know, even if you have not experienced it first-hand, that women get paid less than men for the same work—a mere 82 cents for every dollar earned by men of all races.[3] As if that wasn't upsetting on its own, when women enter traditionally male-dominated jobs, wages go down,[4] and when unemployed men enter traditionally female-dominated jobs, they earn more than the women do.[5]

For many years, women were shut out of jobs. Teaching, retail, banking, nursing, care work—that's the work we were allowed to do. Even then, once we married, it was assumed we'd become mothers and thus many companies preemptively gave us the boot.

And so the whole system was set up to make women unable to financially look after themselves.

It's beyond the scope of this book to go through the history of how women have been excluded from higher education and careers, and even the more recent history of how the coronavirus pandemic sent millions of women out of paid work. But we do need to acknowledge that even today, girls are still being fed damaging stereotypes that have lasting implications. And Boomer women, like me, and Gen Xers are, at midlife and older, living with the harsh realities of those stereotypes.

It's not a new trope that girls are thought to be bad at math, but even I could subtract the cost of living from my minimum-wage salary and see that it was not a very sustainable model. And I wasn't even all that bad in math: I scored 100 percent on my tenth-grade math midterm, which resulted in a friendship after a classmate approached me at the bus stop and asked, "Hey, you're the kid who got 100 on the math midterm, right?" Math may matter in more ways than we give it credit for.

While the narratives around women, math, and money aren't related to midlife per se, the messages we grow up with raise their ugly heads in our romantic relationships and at midlife and later, when women often suffer the worst financially. Some, like me, may have dialed back paying work to be at home to raise children and then struggle to get back into the workplace; others quit altogether, sometimes willingly and other times out of necessity because of the high costs of childcare. Some have to leave their paid work to care-give a spouse, sibling, or parent, or in an increasing number of cases, to raise their grandchildren. Some, like me, find themselves divorced at midlife, or widowed. Some may be happily single and then a financial hit happens—an illness, a recession, a pandemic, furloughs, or layoffs. Some may have lost their job and are unable to find a new one because of ageism. Some have worked hard all their lives and are still struggling as they eye retirement because all women, but especially Black women and other women of color, Native American women, disabled women, and often queer and trans women—who face even more discrimination because of their gender, sexuality, race, and disability—make less than White hetero men. And the ramifications of that are huge and lifelong.

Society has long set up women to be financially dependent on men and then labels us gold diggers if we marry someone wealthier, especially if he's much older, and accuses us of "walking away" with our former husband's money if we divorce, "soaking" or "bleeding" them dry, ignoring the fact that those wives helped create that worth with their paid or unpaid labor.[6] We weren't even able to have access to our own bank accounts, credit cards, and mortgages unless we had a man as a co-signer until the mid-1970s, no matter our relationship status or income, when the laws were changed, thanks in huge part to the efforts of the late Supreme Court Justice Ruth Bader Ginsberg.[7] I know the 1970s may seem like an eternity ago, but it's not; it's my generation, and as a younger Boomer—part of what's considered Generation Jones—I am not "that" old!

While we have come far from that as more women have graduated from college, landed great jobs, busted through glass ceilings, started businesses, secured venture capital funds, and leaned in until we've practically fallen over, many of us still work in gendered workplaces and are expected to do the bulk of the family caregiving, and thus are not financially where we need to be to face what's ahead of us as we age.

It isn't so much that women don't want to know about money; it's more that women get different messages about it from early on, mostly to be careful with it and to save it, not how to invest and grow it.[8] And we do save it, much more than men do.[9] There's nothing wrong with saving and spending judiciously, but that alone will not help us be able to live a good life as we age.

Why would society want to continue to keep women in the dark about money? In what way does that benefit anyone? It certainly doesn't benefit women; in fact, it greatly impacts us negatively. As Beyoncé says, money equals power and if women have money, they also have power. Powerful women can be scary to many men. Sadly, all too often, women are afraid of their own power.

Women's problems with money have almost nothing to do with money per se, and "everything to do with their fear of or ambivalence about power," says financial author Barbara Huson. "[T]he best way to erode our power is to neglect our money or underearn because you cannot possibly play full out if you're drowning in debt, struggling to make ends meet."[10]

What if we got different messages about money, savings, and investing? What if we were expected to be financially savvy and independent? What if we didn't defer to our male romantic partners because they may be older or we believe they're smarter about such things? What if we weren't raised to believe that having a spouse is a financial plan? What if we learned how to be confident about all things financial? What would we do differently with our money? How might that impact our relationships? How would that change when, how, and why we retire, and what our old age looks like?

Thankfully, it's never too late, the financially savvy among us say.

OUR RELATIONSHIP WITH MONEY

First, it's important to explore our emotional relationship with money. I'll start.

I grew up in a solidly middle-class household with frugal parents—products of the Depression and the Holocaust—who paid cash for everything, owned four cars in their sixty-one-year marriage, and ripped paper napkins in half to make them last longer and reused them if only slightly stained. (I did not realize other families didn't do this until much later in life, and I still feel guilty using a whole paper napkin.)

At one point my father stopped buying his favorite blueberry muffins from the wonderful German bakery in town in protest because the price increased a dime and the amount of blueberries slightly decreased.

Although my mother sewed her own clothes from Vogue patterns and European fabric—that woman had style!—as well as clothes for my sister and me (and our Barbie dolls), she liked beautiful things and was a shopper, but always in search of a deal. I will never forget the time she bought my sister and me six pairs of shoes each because they were on sale. One was a neon lime green patent leather sandal with a daisy on the top, and I'd like to go back in time and tell young me, "This is *not* a good look!"

My dad was thrifty, but also a big believer in the stock market. He never relied on a broker's advice; he followed his own gut and brains and did really well. But he never taught his daughters anything about the stock market, although to his credit he did help me invest in Treasury bills back when they paid pretty decent interest. But my parents, like many parents of Boomer kids, expected their daughters to get married in their twenties, and their husbands would take care of financial stuff. Why bother their pretty little heads with such matters?

It would seem, then, that I was a poster child for the narrative about women, that we're bad with financial matters.

"Financial avoidance is a recurring narrative among women and wives, often passed down from previous generations," writes author and financial journalist Farnoosh Torabi, host of the *So Money* podcast.[11]

So, I didn't grow up with a fully rounded view of money, savings, investing, and taking financial risks. As much as I thought I didn't really care all that much about money, I actually care about money a lot. Every decision I have made—from choosing to shop at discount clothing or consignment stores, to often ordering the cheapest (or close to it) item on a menu when dining out, to skipping events I really wanted to go to because the tickets were too expensive—is based on my relationship with money. Because I have one, even if I didn't realize it, and so do you.

And as a woman, that relationship is no doubt complicated, as psychotherapist Kate Levinson details in her book *Emotional Currency: A Woman's Guide to Building a Healthy Relationship With Money.*

"We live in a culture that until very recently thought women's financial place was to be dependent on men. It taught, and often legally required, women to rely on their fathers, husbands, brothers, sons and financial experts to handle their financial concerns," she writes. "For centuries women were kept away from money, even when it was our own. This marginalization of women in the legal and public spheres of money contributed to our developing a strong interior relationship with it."[12]

Is it any wonder that women, despite the huge financial gains we have made in the workplace in recent years, aren't always as savvy at dealing with money? We were never expected to be. No one wanted us to be. And while times have changed, many of us at midlife and older are behind in preparing financially for our older selves. Way behind.

THE DIVORCE (MONEY) DIET

When I divorced the second time, after years of working part time so I could be at home for our sons—an arrangement my husband and I agreed to because he was more established in his career and made more money than I did—I began to realize money's value. Once again, despite going back to the workforce full time, I didn't have a lot. I was in my fifties when I finally made the salary my father made as a mechanical engineer when I was a child. For reference, my car cost a few thousand dollars more than the house I grew up in. And now I had two children to support.

As they say, it wasn't pretty. I bounced checks all the time in those days.

Like many Boomers, I divorced at midlife. Although the divorce rate is falling for Millennials and Gen Xers, those now in their thirties and forties, the divorce rate is increasing for people fifty and older, according to the Pew Research Center.[13] And for the middle-aged now-divorced moms who gave up or dialed back their careers to raise children as I did, they are realizing just how much they have given up—financially, especially if they weren't fully aware of all the financial goings-on in their marriage.

Shockingly, that is a lot of women. According to a 2021 UBS report, 48 percent of women surveyed by the investment bank and financial services company said their spouse is responsible for all the long-term financial decisions, including investing, and financial and estate planning. And the wives were fine with it. In fact, only 29 percent of Boomer women who defer to their husband say they would like to have more of a say in their financial goings-on, while 58 percent of Gen Xers say the same.[14]

One of those women was Robin Hauser, a San Francisco Bay Area filmmaker who got the idea for her latest documentary, *$avvy*, on how gender norms around money leave women particularly vulnerable, when she was reeling from a divorce after a twenty-five-year marriage. She was fifty at the time.

Despite having an MBA, and a career both in international business and as a stockbroker, Hauser wasn't very hands-on with the family's finances until the divorce forced her. Then she discovered many of her female friends also had little to no part in their family's finances.[15] What was going on, she wondered.

"I'd been thinking about how even really smart educated women just sort of abdicate major financial stuff to the men in our lives. We tend to take a backseat to personal finance," Hauser, who now is in her late fifties, tells me. "Even women who manage their own household and expenses don't necessarily get involved in investing and long-term savings."[16]

Why not? According to the UBS report, women gave a variety of reasons for letting their husbands take charge of the finances; they either don't know where to begin, or they think their husband knows more about such things, or they have other responsibilities, or they don't have much interest, or—this made me pause—they want to be taken care of.

Somehow, they either lost sight of the message of personal financial responsibility, or they never got it. But did they want to hear it?

When longtime journalist Leslie Bennetts published her book *The Feminine Mistake: Are We Giving Up Too Much?*—a plea to moms that they never give up their career and become financially dependent on a romantic partner—it was met with some praise but much more criticism.

Writing in the *New York Times,* book reviewer Eugenie Allen wished that Bennetts had acknowledged that "it's possible for a woman to find deep meaning in a life spent mostly caring for her family. Instead, Bennetts portrays the stay-at-home mother as a financial and emotional drain on her husband; a bad example for their children; and a disappointment to her gender, to society and, worst of all, to herself."[17]

The *New Yorker's* Rebecca Mead pooh-poohed Bennetts's warn-ings of financial devastation by sudden widowhood or divorce, noting that "to some extent such circumstances can be hedged against with insurance policies and the efforts of a decent matrimo-nial lawyer."[18] If that were true for every woman, we wouldn't see such a large percentage of divorcees and widows living in poverty.[19] A stay-at-home mom of two young boys I know became a widow in her early forties when her self-employed contractor husband died suddenly. He had no life insurance policy. As for hiring a "decent matrimonial lawyer," they don't come cheap; not every woman can afford an attorney when hourly rates average $270, but often charge much more.[20] I certainly couldn't.

Bennetts's book came out in March 2007. Nine months later, the Great Recession hit and 69 percent of U.S. men—many of them breadwinners—lost their jobs and, even a decade later, many still hadn't found work.[21] Few at-home wives predicted that, and many who found "deep meaning" caring for their family suddenly were forced back into the workplace.

The reverse happened in 2020, when the coronavirus pandemic hit and millions of women lost their jobs or had to cut their hours or quit entirely to oversee children who were doing virtual learning for months. Women overwhelmingly said they struggled to pay bills, their rent or mortgage, and medical care, and were more likely to dip into their retirement money and borrow money from family or friends due to the pandemic.[22] It was promptly called a shecession.[23] Again, who saw this coming except perhaps virologists?

Many predict the coronavirus pandemic will be a huge and long-lasting hit to women's lives and gender equality—perhaps even sending women back ten years or more.[24] And scientists predict more pandemics ahead, and all the financial ramifications of that.

Beyond our financial struggles, quarantining for weeks on end put a huge strain on many couples, and the result could be a spike in divorce post-pandemic. Other women became widows due to COVID-19, or had a spouse who became too sick to work after being intubated or from other long-term effects.[25]

None of this was in our life plans. It certainly wasn't in mine. Still, this will make women—who get paid less than men, tend to move in and out of the workforce more than men, and live longer than men—even more vulnerable, especially since the share of mothers who do not work outside the home has risen over the past decade.[26]

Even the ones who do work outside the home had a much harder time finding work after the Great Recession than men. All of which points to the need for women to be financially savvy and independent, whether they're partnered or not.

As Bennetts tells me, "That blueprint we give women isn't working for us anymore, the blueprint that says one person can kind of resign from the responsibility of taking charge of her own life and hand that over to someone else, that is not a viable blueprint for the length and the challenges of the typical adult life in the 21st century. . . . The pandemic is just another version of what I was writing about. You can't necessarily in the long run count on anybody but yourself so you need to take responsibility for your own life, you need to plan for various eventualities, some of which may not be the ones you want, and figure out how you can survive them. Because it's a long journey and life presents a lot of challenges if you live long enough."

PLEASE TAKE CARE OF ME

In describing how she went from being the breadwinner in her first two marriages—not by choice—to being an equal financial partner with her third husband, author Karen Karbo questions if she would have been able to leave her first marriage so easily if she had been financially dependent on her husband.

"It brings up a question that can only be posed uneasily: Is it better for the longevity of a marriage if one party (usually the woman) feels financially trapped?" she writes.[27]

Of course, that is not how women generally view marriage, and it's not how we talk about marriage in general. We marry for love and companionship, and maybe someone to raise children with, right? We don't see it as a financial arrangement (although it historically has been and continues to be) even though nearly 60 percent of married Millennial women say they want to be "taken care of."[28] Being "taken care of" is actually a financial decision, whether you care to look at it that way or not, and not necessarily a wise one.

Karbo understands the feeling, though.

"I still would love to experience life as a pampered princess, at least once. I'd love to be the kind of woman you see in jewelry commercials around the holidays who sits before a fire, a cashmere throw over her knees. Suddenly, her beloved swoops in with a velvet-covered box, bearing some hideous pendant that nevertheless cost real money. I envy this woman because she is so taken with her beloved's generosity. She never says, 'Honey, why did you buy me this piece of crap when you know I need a new crown on my back molar?' . . . I would love to be a woman who is able to indulge in the magical thinking that romance always matters more than money."[29]

Who wouldn't? Even high-earning women can fall victim to that romantic magical thinking. Take model Paulina Porizkova, who thought romance mattered more than money when she married The Cars frontman Ric Ocasek when she was twenty-four and he was forty-five. She was bringing in $6 million a year at the time, an income that could support a very good life for decades.[30]

Like many women, she says she let her husband take care of the financial things—it was that older, wiser man thing. They separated after twenty-eight years of marriage and were on their way to a divorce when Ocasek suddenly died at age seventy-five. That's when Porizkova discovered he'd cut her out of his will, leaving her without any access to their money, even her own earnings, at midlife. Does she blame him? No, she blames herself (although she admits to being a bit pissed off at him, and rightfully so).

"What happened to me, it seemed like it was so easily preventable. And it was based on not misfortune, it was based on my own stupidity," she says. "Now if I had a daughter, any of my goddaughters or granddaughters or any of the young women I know . . . if there's one good thing I could do for them is to let them hear my story of how romance eclipsed any financial thinking and what a bad idea that is."[31]

And yet, hetero men and women of all ages and all ethnicities overwhelmingly believe a man should be the financial provider for his family to be a good husband or partner.[32] That keeps men and women in a highly gendered dynamic.

A 2015 Gallup poll indicates that 56 percent of moms with children under age eighteen would prefer to be at home instead of heading off to work, which could easily be interpreted as women making that choice happily.[33] Not always. As Darlena Cunha, a Millennial mother of two, writes in *Time*, without paid maternity leave and affordable childcare, and with "unsupportive or nonexistent family policies," and that darn wage gap, many mothers have little choice.[34] Perhaps that's why a third of at-home mothers live in poverty.[35]

Shockingly, 46 percent of women who don't have young children and aren't working also say they prefer to be a homemaker—aka "taken care of." Not to say that the work involved in keeping a home and family cared for is not essential. It is. It just often leaves women in financially precarious situations when they least can afford to be. (Actually, there's never a good time to be in a financially precarious situation, is there?)

As we saw in chapter 4, we get bombarded with messages about looking young, thin, and beautiful, and so we women spend a lot of our money, not to mention our time and energy, buying products and having procedures to achieve that to various degrees of success. That might be OK if we also got the same amount of messages about doing other things with our money, like savings, investing, and planning for a happily retired and financially secure future self. But we generally don't. And even if we know we should look after our money, we often doubt ourselves.

Maybe it's because there's a substantial number of women who grew up feeling uncomfortable with math. Maybe you didn't get a Teen Talk Barbie, the one who declared, "Math class is tough!" as a young girl, but you might have heard your mother say she was never any good at math or had a female teacher who seemed somewhat anxious whenever she taught math. Researchers found that in both cases, a girl's achievement in the subject slips almost immediately.[36] If math seems "tough," knowing how to manage your money isn't going to be easier.

According to one study, women are less willing than men to manage their own retirement account investments, even though both men and women agree that being able to manage their investments by themselves is a huge plus. "The decision to not make decisions is a problem that compounds the disadvantages that women already face when building their retirements savings: women are paid less than men and often work fewer years, due to taking time out of the workforce for child-rearing."[37] And remember, we often live longer than men, so have a much longer retirement.

Women often retire at the same time that their husband does, perhaps to travel or indulge in long-deferred dreams together. But because women typically are younger than their husbands, retiring early—often at their peak earning years—robs them of substantial

Chapter 7

future earnings and more Social Security benefits. "Unless married couples have other assets—from savings, for example—women's younger retirement age means they have less wealth to live on during their remaining life together, and during any subsequent divorce or widowhood," notes Nicole Maestas, who leads the National Bureau of Economic Research's Retirement and Disability Research Center.[38]

Clearly this is a conversation couples need to have but often don't have, leaving a lot of unhappiness on both sides.[39] Still, since women are impacted the most, it would seem like having her decide when to retire would be a smart form of financial self-care.

"Being able to take care of yourself today financially isn't the same thing as being financially independent or financially empowered," says sociologist Marianne Cooper, of Stanford University's Women's Leadership Innovation Lab. "Being financially independent means being in a position to take care of yourself for life and to afford the life you want, independent of whether you end up sharing it with someone or not."[40]

Black women often face a unique narrative that impacts them financially—the Strong Black Woman Syndrome, writes financial coach and author Kara Stevens. All too often that syndrome demands a type of "financial martyrdom" that puts everyone else's needs, from their adult children or grandchildren to their community, above their own. "The Strong Black Woman Syndrome is a racist and sexist archetype created to emotionally and financially marginalize Black women," she writes. "It keeps Black women far from emotional happiness and financial wellness, thus limiting access to their full humanity."[41]

Financial journalist Jennifer L. Barrett urges women to think like they are their family's breadwinner, which is the title of her 2021 book, *Think Like a Breadwinner: A Wealth-Building Manifesto for Women Who Want to Earn More (and Worry Less),* even if they actually are. And the number of female breadwinners is growing all the time; 41 percent of moms are the sole or main breadwinners for their families. Black mothers are much more likely than White or Hispanic moms to be their family's sole breadwinner, a reality for decades.[42]

Barrett learned the hard way when the startup her husband worked for, which paid much more than her job, went belly up, and he eventually landed at a much lower-paying job. "It hadn't occurred to me that the man I married, who had an MBA and a better-paying job when we got engaged, might not always be in a position to take the lead in our financial lives. Or maybe I didn't want to consider that possibility because I wasn't sure I could (or wanted to) fill that role," she writes.[43]

Is it wrong for women to want to rely on marriage as their financial plan?

Not necessarily, says University of Auckland emeritus professor Maureen Baker, who studies social policy issues that impact women and families. A long-time partner who brings in the bucks is "the most effective way that women can protect themselves in retirement," she says. "It's logical, it's not stupid, because women on their own cannot earn the same."[44]

I'd actually much prefer to earn the same as men, quite honestly.

Beyond impacting our future financial selves, earning less money has huge ramifications for our health: women who get paid less are at far greater risk for developing depression and anxiety than women who are paid the same as men.[45]

I'm not sure girls still grow up hearing, "It's just as easy to fall in love with a rich man as it is to fall in love with a poor one," as I did, but I'm pretty sure there aren't many parents who encourage their sons to "marry up."

Still, Baker says, women should be prepared for the unexpected — things like divorce, illness, a spouse's unemployment, a disability — by making her own money and controlling her own savings.

But even being the breadwinner doesn't protect a woman.

My friend supported her family of four as a doctor, and because she hated dealing with anything financial, she let her husband take care of it. They lived a cushy life with a large home and a pool in a wealthy city in the San Francisco Bay Area. When they were divorcing, she discovered he had committed financial infidelity — it has nothing to do with sexual shenanigans, but things like hiding money, incurring debt, and having credit cards without a spouse's knowledge, and it happens a lot. She was livid. He ended up with the family home, and she had to start all over again in her early fifties. Understandably, she regrets not keeping tabs on their money.

Actually, older women of all races and ethnicities have more than a few regrets when it comes to money, according to a 2020 report by Merrill Lynch, *Women & Financial Wellness*. Some wish they had chosen a higher-paying career and didn't pile on the credit card debt. The biggest regret, however, was that they hadn't invested more. But working against them is a lack of knowledge and confidence in investing.[46]

That was my reality, too.

Actually, I never had any money to invest until my parents died and I inherited some stocks. Not anywhere near enough to retire on, but more than I ever imagined I'd have. I was in my mid-fifties at the time, with a 401(k) that wouldn't have lasted me a year. I bought the family house from my husband when we divorced because I wanted my boys to finish high school in their family home, but I never imagined I'd be able to hold onto it. I qualified for a five-year interest-only loan back in the day when you didn't have to show your income—they would have laughed—just that you were employed. But I had a rental unit in the house that covered half of my mortgage, and we had a lot of equity in the house. This was the smartest decision I ever made, after having my children, and I know owning and holding on to a home isn't within reach for many people.

I hired a financial advisor, not to tell me where to put my money but to help me strategize various scenarios of what I would be willing to do if I got laid off—a constant fear in the ever-shrinking world of media—or could no longer work due to an illness or disability. She helped me figure out how long I would need to keep working before I could retire, assuming no calamity like an earthquake or a fire put a huge dent in my finances. How does seventy sound? I'm exhausted thinking about it.

So, I started learning about the stock market and investments, and I began hustling. I amped up my freelance writing, rented out a room in my house through Airbnb in addition to my rental unit—anything that I could monetize, I monetized because I can't live on my salary alone, which is distressingly considered "very low income" in the San Francisco Bay Area. While I have no regrets about not choosing a higher-paying career because I have loved working at newspapers and covering my community, I absolutely wish I had negotiated a better salary from the start and been much more assertive about asking for raises.

I actually have asked for raises over the years but didn't get them. I'm not alone, a new study indicates. Women ask for raises as much as men do, but while 20 percent of the men who ask actually get a raise, just 15 percent of women do. As the researchers note, "While that may sound like a modest difference, over a lifetime it really adds up."[47] I figure I've lost more than $100,000. Now you can see why so many midlife and older women live in poverty, especially if they're divorced.[48]

For someone who never cared about money, I started to care. I finally got the message: I and I alone am responsible for my own finances, and if I ever hope to retire—and I do, hopefully before seventy!—I had better get on it ASAP.

Like for Robin Hauser and countless other women, my divorce was the wake-up call.

MINIMAL STUFF, MAXIMUM MONEY

Whatever you may think about uber-successful momager-mogul Kris Jenner, the brains behind the reality TV series *Keeping Up With the Kardashians,* it probably isn't that she's bad with money. But the mother of six—Khloé, Kim, Kourtney, and Rob Kardashian, and Kylie and Kendall Jenner—says she knew nothing about the family finances when she divorced her first husband, the late Robert Kardashian. When a friend asked her how much she paid her gardener, she had no idea. "I was embarrassed that I didn't know. I woke up one day to responsibilities that I hadn't had the day before. And I needed to figure it out," she tells the *Wall Street Journal.* "I felt such an enormous sense of accomplishment to be able to figure it all out and pay my own bills and make my own money and do my own taxes. And there were times when I didn't have a lot of money, but I was very organized."[49]

Divorce evidently does more than just boost a woman's libido, as we saw in chapter 2; it forces women to look into the mirror and say, "Please take care of me" to themselves.

When Gen X single mom Christine Platt married in her thirties, she eagerly set about decorating their newly purchased 2,500-square-foot house and indulging in things that a young, hard-working and successful couple clearly "deserved" (her word) to have. Platt, the managing director at American University's Antiracist Research & Policy Center, admits she took pride in her overflowing closets and drawers, embracing an "I-buy-what-I-want-because-I-deserve-it-especially-if-it's-on-sale" mindset. Bargain shopping became her escape. I can relate.

Then her marriage of six years ended in 2016, and she found herself back in the 630-square-foot one-bedroom, one-bathroom Washington, D.C., condo she bought as a single Black woman and attorney. Freed from her marriage and from her "stuff," her flirtations of becoming a minimalist suddenly had to become reality. She had no choice.[50] Now she helps other people, especially Black women, change that "I deserve it" philosophy on her Afrominimalist website. Her minimalism is informed by the history, culture, and beauty of the African diaspora, she writes in her 2021 book, *The Afrominimalist's Guide to Living with Less.* That was not something she found in the mainstream minimalism movement, which means it missed some important realities of systemic oppression and how many Black people's "inherited beliefs have a profound influence on our relationship with money and ownership."[51]

Platt believes once we better understand how those beliefs have impacted our own lives and explore our "I deserve this" purchases, we can make different, hopefully better, financial decisions in the future.[52]

Minimalism isn't about saving money per se, but it's a philosophy that works particularly well for women at midlife and beyond. Sometimes, we're forced into living frugally, either because we've lost a job and can't find a new one—a situation many women find themselves in at midlife, thanks to ageism—or we had to quit our job because of health or care-giving reasons. That's a whole different reality than making conscious choices of how we want to spend our time, money, and energy, as Platt has.

The myth is that men make money and are inherently savvy about it while women are better at spending it. Although research indicates that men are just as likely to splurge as women are, women get the bulk of blame for it. Of course we would.[53]

On her *Smart Living 365* blog and in her book *Rightsizing: A Smart Living 365 Guide to Reinventing Retirement,* author Kathy Gottberg promotes the idea of rightsizing. It isn't just about the size of your house, although that is what people often think of; it's more about consciously choosing a life that fits who you are and brings you the most peace, joy, and contentment. And it starts with learning how to manage your expenses and income, she says. Among those are messages we hear over and over and often ignore, to our financial peril: living below our means, not spending money we don't have, not buying things as investments that don't actually generate income, and honestly assessing what you think you need and what you actually need (they are not the same).[54]

The pandemic showed many women how little we actually need to live, not only all the beauty routines and procedures we spend a huge amount of money on, as we saw in chapter 4, but also how we could happily exist in yoga pants, PJs, and bare feet and without shampooing or showering for days on end if we had the luxury of working from home. If you're like me, you saw a bit more money in your bank account if you weren't ordering left and right online.

I am not a minimalist, but the pandemic did make me look at just how much I had been consuming. I felt embarrassed and a little stupid. I had to ask myself why was I working so hard only to end up with so much stuff I really didn't need when I could have put that money to much better use, like for my retirement or for something I really want to do, like travel or take art classes or go to a concert even if the tickets are pricey. Yes, I should have spent that $252 to see Jackson Browne, a heartthrob of mine when I was a teen, play a benefit concert at the legendary Sweetwater Music Hall in 2018.

Actually, I had already begun to think about overconsumption when I cleaned out my parents' 2,500-square-foot Florida condo nearly twelve years ago. My mother had gorgeous clothes with the price tags still attached (my dad's clothes took up less than a tenth of the room in their spacious walk-in closet), and her "special dishes"—one of three sets of dishes she owned—looked like they had never been used. They had been, but about once a month, if that, when they entertained. The dishes brought pennies on the dollar when I sold them. I know they brought my mother joy to use, but they might have brought her a lot more joy if she used them every day. When I returned to my San Francisco Bay Area home, I immediately started purging.

Not to say that all women start hoarding as we age, but research indicates that many of us do, mostly driven by an inability to let go of our stuff. (For the record, older men become hoarders just as easily, so it's not just on us.)[55] But we have to start accumulating that stuff in the first place. If we're like Platt, many of us have heard "you deserve it" and "you're worth it" messages for years. Single women are especially targeted around Valentine's Day. Don't have a boo? Don't worry! You can "survive" the day—like it's a disease!—by showing yourself some self-love. Too bad most of the self-love advice has us treating ourselves in ways that we'll still be paying for the next Valentine's Day, either as charges on our credit cards or extra pounds on our body.

Money is intertwined with things like self-worth, abundance and deprivation, protection, autonomy and dependency, and envy, Levinson writes, and that's what we bring into our relationships, as do our partners. There's a reason why money is one of the top issues couples fight about. For many men, money is all about power and status; for many women it's a mix of "guilt, pain, danger, and fear as well as love, self-worth, nurturance and security."[56]

Women also tend to use it for different reasons. "The real goal is to help others," financial author Barbara Stanny says in her conversation with financial journalist Farnoosh Torabi.[57]

Not to brag about women, but women actually do use their money to help others, according to a survey by the Economist Intelligence Unit. High-earning women, especially Gen X and younger women, say that making a difference in society and benefitting others is often a factor in their financial decisions. "It is apparent that getting more assets in the hands of more women is good for society at large," writes Angie O'Leary, of RBC Wealth Management, which commissioned the study.[58]

I love that women are drawn to building up their community and helping others. I think that's being incredibly good with money.

Now, we just need to get more women to help themselves.

Tired of the narrative that women are bad with money and that if we're poor or haven't invested or saved, it's somehow our fault, many women are now raising their voices and trying to get other women to raise theirs to talk openly and honestly about money. Some are appealing to the Latinx community, like Gen Xer Beatriz Acevedo, who co-founded a digital financial-technology company, SUMA Wealth, in 2020. Latinas were among the hardest hit financially during the pandemic.

Author and financial coach Kara Stevens, aka the Frugal Feminista, seeks to help Black women take control of their finances and grow their wealth. Wall Street veteran Sallie Krawcheck co-founded the investment platform Ellevest in 2014 primarily to help all women become financially literate.

Others are targeting Millennials, like twenty-nine-year-old Haley Sacks, aka Mrs. Dow Jones, a self-described "financial pop star" who offers entertaining and easy to understand lessons on all things finance to thousands of her followers on YouTube, Twitter, and TikTok.

Millennial women have thankfully gotten more financial education in high school, college, or on the job than Boomer women and Gen X women, and the gap between their financial literacy and Millennial men's is closing. That's promising.[59]

But where does that leave women who are at midlife and older right now?

Some of us might be behind, but it's not too late.

Once we strip away the narratives and see how they've hurt us financially, we can drown out the noise about how bad we are at managing money, question ourselves on how buying into those narratives have led us to where we are financially at this moment, and start getting real about what we want moving forward.

"The truth is if you can add and subtract, you can manage your finances. You can ask questions. You can educate yourself. No one knows your needs better than you," says Janet Lombardi, who details in her book, *Bankruptcy: A Love Story*, how her husband of twenty-five years drained all their financial accounts, unbeknownst to her, while also bilking a client before being carted off to jail.[60] You bet she's managing her money on her own now.

The pandemic has left a lot of people anxious about their finances, especially women. WealthiHer, a network founded by women that seeks to help women grow and protect their wealth, surveyed more than 2,000 men and women in 2020 to discover how they've fared during the pandemic. Not so great. More than 70 percent of women have seen their financial plans disrupted, causing them to feel less financially secure, while 59 percent had to stop contributing to their retirement plans.[61]

Even before the pandemic, older women had a lot of anxiety about retiring, mostly the rising cost of goods, potential reduction in their Social Security or Medicare benefits, health care costs, and not properly estimating their future expenses and their ability to pay for them.[62]

Talking about all things financial with other women may be helpful, notes Stacy Francis, president and chief executive officer of Francis Financial. She gathers monthly with other women to do just that. "We don't necessarily talk about numbers. We talk about our relationship with money, we learn from each other. It is really powerful."[63]

Ultimately, however, our future financial self is in our own hands. As Farnoosh Torabi writes, no one cares more about your money than you do, not your romantic partner and not even your financial advisor. "The depth of pain and excitement around your money is yours and yours only. The difference between making money and losing it is in your hands, which is pretty empowering. This is a major financial philosophy of mine. It encourages me to speak up, ask questions, negotiate, and take responsible steps to protect and grow my hard-earned money."[64]

And if that doesn't inspire you to start planning for your future self's financial future, consider this: Being financially secure played a big role in shaping Boomers' attitude about menopause. It lessened whatever anxiety they may have had about losing their fertility and attractiveness at midlife.[65]

Guess you can call that their "f*ck-you" money. You can have that, too.

THINGS TO THINK ABOUT

What is your relationship with money?
What do you wish you knew about financial matters?
Did you grow up believing you were bad at math and money?
Have you taken responsibility for your own finances?
In what ways do you feel prepared or not for your future
    financial self?

8

✝

A Love Letter to Women

See your life in the long distance.

—Norma Kamali[1]

In her book *The Genius of Women: From Overlooked to Changing the World,* which highlights the achievements of women who have long been ignored, undermined, and overlooked, author Janice Kaplan wonders what the world would be like if women had the same early support and encouragement in developing their potential as men have. What would the rest of their life look like, and how would their fulfilled potential benefit society?

We'll never know, but we can imagine. Many of us have experienced being ignored, undermined, and overlooked, if not in our youth, then it awaits us at midlife, or so we are led to believe.

Oh joy!

It would be easy to point the finger at men, but it's not all men's fault—although can we please acknowledge that they started it? But we take it from there. Women, Kaplan says, "buy into the system. We assume the male-dominated water in which we are swimming is the only possible environment, so we don't allow ourselves to jump out and sample fresh air. We undermine our own achievements and don't expect to do as well as men. We scare ourselves away from success long before anyone else sends us away."[2]

I know that I have been guilty of that.

151

I thought about her words while I was researching and writing this book, applying it to the harmful narratives we've heard about aging as a woman and how we "buy into the system." Once we hit midlife, society makes us feel ignored and overlooked, but way before then we live in fear of aging and thus spend a lot of time, money, and physical and mental energy contorting ourselves to seem anything but "old."

What if things were different? What if girls grew up in a world that didn't place such an emphasis on their youth and beauty; that encouraged and supported them to believe that they are complete on their own, without the need for validation from others; that didn't promote finding romantic love, especially if it seemed like a way to be "taken care of," over developing and nurturing non-romantic friendships across ages, races, genders, beliefs; that equipped them with knowledge for financial success, beyond just paying them what they're worth (if they even get there); that didn't set them on a path to internalize the ageist, sexist system that hurts them throughout their lives, including their future selves? A world that stopped giving men carte blanche to write the narratives about women's lives.

Is it a tall order? Perhaps. Can we, as eldresses, as actor Frances McDormand would like to be known as she ages, help make that happen? We can certainly try. I believe we must.

Of course, that means first questioning and sorting out our own possibly conflicted feelings of aging as a woman in the twenty-first century. My hope is that after reading this book, you are getting closer to that point. My research has made me much more conscious about how I think, talk, and write about older women—including myself. It's too late for how I thought of my beloved singer-songwriter, but I'm much more aware now. When one of my free-lance columnists included a sexist and ageist quote, something about little old ladies playing music to their cats, in one of his columns, I took out the quote. It added nothing of substance to the column and just repeated a clichéd, condescending stereotype that I'm not going to allow in my newspaper section. Or accept in my life.

And that's how we change the narratives, one woman at a time consciously choosing to think and act differently about aging. We'll never be able to address the rampant ageism around us and offer a better world for the next generation of women if we don't.

Remember, that's how foot binding stopped in China; the women who perpetuated the crippling mark of beauty finally said, *no more.*

As we explored in chapter 7, moms and female teachers who express anxiety about math set the stage for their daughters and female students' achievement to plummet almost immediately; so, too, do our thoughts, words, and actions when it comes to aging. What are young women—and young men, for that matter—absorbing from us?

Take journalist Rebecca Knight's essay "Balancing feminism with caring about what I look like" in the online parenting publication *Motherwell.* Knight describes herself as a "feminist mom," yet her story illustrates how young women, in this case her twelve-year-old daughter, are watching us, feminist or not, and getting mixed messages.

"I've raised my daughter to believe that a preoccupation with one's appearance is at best trivial, at worst an affront to womankind. But I am a traitor to the cause. . . . It's too late for me. At this point, I've already fallen prey to the immense pressure that society puts on women to try to look a certain way," she writes. "I may be a liberated, modern woman, but I am also more than a little bit skin-deep. It's not too late for my daughter, however. The idea of self-acceptance—even in the face of the all-powerful beauty industrial complex—needn't feel like a scam for her. She doesn't need to abide by impossible standards."[3]

No, she doesn't need to abide by those exhausting standards. But she most likely will because in the twelve years that she's been alive, and all the years to follow, she will have watched her feminist mother give in to societal pressure to "try to look a certain way." And that "certain way" is to not look old. It's a classic example of "do as I say, not as I do," or, in some circles, "OK Boomer."

Ageism starts early—as early as childhood—and as young people get a sense of what growing older looks like in a world that prioritizes youth, it's no wonder that aging seems like something to fear, especially for a woman.

A CNN article in 2021 documents a disturbing trend: more teenage girls are obsessing about "premature aging" and turning to products that "focus on science and proof," as if science, or any beauty product or procedure, has found a way to avoid aging (FYI, they have not). It prompted one clinical psychologist to call that kind of thinking "hopelessness about the future"—their own future.[4]

"I just don't like the look of wrinkles. And that's probably because society has conditioned me not to like the look of wrinkles. . . . So I'll prevent it if I can," fifteen-year-old Kennedy Hack-Juman tells CNN.[5]

So, yes, young women are paying close attention to what people are saying—and doing—about aging, at least the physical aspects of aging. And that is drowning out the voices of women like Frances McDormand and others who refuse to buy in to the system and focusing on one small aspect of getting older over much more pressing realities.

Yet, as we age, research says we surprisingly become less anxious about getting older. Whatever ageist attitudes we have about growing old change as we age. We may have had feelings about turning forty and then we hit forty and it's not so bad. We don't feel all that different inside, even if the outside looks different. Same when we turn fifty and sixty. Unfortunately, we also, distressingly, start to develop more stereotypes and prejudices about aging. In fact, older people tend to be more prejudiced about people in their own age group than younger people are, as they try to differentiate themselves from the "oldest old" people. Go figure![6]

Clearly, we have some work to do.

Anna Rosa Donizzetti, of the University of Naples Federico II's humanities department, suggests society needs to institute preventive programs to teach people about the aging process, which is completely natural and lifelong. Knowledge is power, after all. "Making an intervention among the youngest populations will guarantee to all of society's future generations that they are no longer gripped by anxiety about what the future holds for them," she writes.[7]

That would certainly help.

That said, no amount of preventive programs and interventions are going to override what young women observe and internalize while watching how the older women around them, whether they're their mothers, aunties, neighbors, coworkers, or friends, deal with aging. And if a twelve-year-old watches her mother freak out about wrinkles and gray hair while telling her that a woman's beauty doesn't matter, well, good luck with that. Young people are incredibly good at sniffing out hypocrisy.

Does that mean that women should stop getting Botox, dying their gray hair, slathering on anti-aging serums, and doing whatever other routines they do to keep themselves looking young? Not necessarily.

In her book *Face: One Square Foot of Skin,* actor Justine Bateman makes a case against cosmetic surgery. She's out to convince women that there's nothing wrong with their face—they don't need to cut it up and inject toxins into it.

I admire her goal, but I don't believe in telling women what they "should" or "shouldn't" do. Don't women get enough of those messages as it is?

I'm more in alignment with Sesali Bowen, aka @BadFatBlackGirl, whom we met in chapter 4. The new narratives about aging should make room for all types of beauty and bodies—including women who tinker with their face, hair, body, nails, whatever. If that's what makes them feel good, I am all for it—with a caveat.

What we really need is for women of all ages to start having honest conversations about not just what they perceive as the negatives of aging as a woman in this world, but also the ways that getting older has made them stronger, more resilient, more open-minded, more accepting. To share the fears they had about getting older, and what they did, or didn't do, to work through their fears and whether what they feared ever actually materialized. Not a list of regrets, but the things they've learned along the way. Not that they will have the answers or the "secret," or that what worked for them will work for everyone, but more to encourage a curiosity about what we're told about aging versus how women actually experience it. How they have moved toward "becoming."

If young women go along with the current narratives about older women, then they'll no doubt have to live with the very same narratives themselves when they hit their forties, fifties, and beyond. And spend years being impacted by their harmful messages.

"I think reflecting on aging can help to build bridges across generations of women, once we see ageism itself as a common enemy," says Lynne Segal, a professor of psychology and gender studies at Birkbeck University of London, and author of *Out of Time: The Pleasures and Perils of Aging.* "The essence of ageism is its repudiations of human frailty and dependence. Yet we all depend upon routine forms of care, recognition and support from others throughout our lives. We flourish in and through our relations to others, and the responsibilities this places on us to care for one another. And this in turn means, as feminists have always known, that we must address

all the ways that the work of caring has been and remains undervalued. Especially in these times of growing environmental danger,
admitting our shared human vulnerabilities can help to unite us in
revaluing all practices that promote forms of flourishing—human,
non-human and planetary."[8]

Journalist and author Caitlin Moran, in her mid-forties, would
like to see the same. "We don't sell the idea of being an older woman
to younger women. We don't show that you are still the same bril-
liant, clever, funny person—and now you've also got systems, you
can cope."[9]

Yes to all that.

We have an opportunity to create new narratives of aging as a
woman, ones that value women at all stages of life, not just youth.
The world is getting very close to being populated by more old
people than young people—it's going to be impossible to ignore
us. There's power in numbers. And just as there will be many more
old people than young people in the near future, they are also more
likely to live longer lives, so the world will be old for a very long
time. And since women live longer than men do, a long-lived society is inevitably a "feminized" society.[10]

The slogan that came out of the 1970s lesbian separatist moment,
"The future is female," looks like it's going to actually be true.

How do we want to spend those years? Certainly not being held
back by sexist, ageist narratives.

Rainesford Stauffer, author of *An Ordinary Age: Finding Your Way
in a World That Expects Exceptional,* appreciates how new narratives
would help her Millennial generation and the ones that will follow.
The traditional markers of adulthood—graduating college, career,
marriage, children, homeownership—have either been postponed
or are out of reach for her generation and Gen Xers. That, no doubt,
will impact their future older selves.

"The ageist mentality that only one period counts in our lives,
above all the others, feeds systems that thrive on us never feeling
like we're enough—until we're too much, or 'too old,'" Stauffer
writes. "Maybe if we embraced aging as part of how we grow up
and make our way in the world, we'd find value in all of life's
stages, and thwart the pressure-cooker sensation that we're running
out of time. We won't have 'done it all' by 25. We'll end up with a
fuller life, instead."[11]

Aging is indeed how we make our way in the world, from the second we're born. It's the only way to get us to our future self, with all her wrinkles, sagging, crepey skin, age spots, and gray hair if we are lucky to live that long. Who is that future woman? How do you want her to live? How do you want the world to treat her? What might help her feel valued, loved, vibrant, financially secure, cared for?

If you've ever looked back at yourself as a young girl or young woman, not to give her advice, but to hold her with compassion and kindness, as if she were your BFF, then why not grant your future self the same?

You get to write your future self's story, starting now. My wish for you is that it's a story with a truly happy ending.

Notes

INTRODUCTION

1. "Age discrimination laws don't protect older women as they do older men," University at Buffalo, June 18, 2020, *ScienceDaily*, www.sciencedaily .com/releases/2020/06/200618120157.htm.

2. "Hollywood Diversity Report 2020," *UCLA College Social Sciences*, 2020, https://socialsciences.ucla.edu/hollywood-diversity-report-2020).

3. Andrea Mandell, "Where are real portrayals of women over 50 on screen? New study highlights dearth of leading roles," *USA Today*, October 27, 2020, https://www.usatoday.com/story/entertainment/movies /2020/10/27/women-over-50-losing-out-major-movie-roles-study-finds /6048202002.

4. Laura Carstensen, *A Long Bright Future: Happiness, Health, and Financial Security in an Age of Increased Longevity* (New York: Harmony, 2009) 23.

5. Jenkins, Jo Ann, *Disrupt Aging: A Bold New Path to Living Your Best Life at Every Age* (New York: PublicAffairs, 2016) 40.

6. Molly Andrews, "Ageful and proud," *Ageing and Society*, 20, 6 (November 2000): 791–95.

7. Vivian Sobchack, "Scary Women: Cinema, Surgery, and Special Effects," in *Figuring Age: Women, Bodies, Generations*, ed. Kathleen Woodward (Indiana: Indiana University Press, 1999) 200–11.

8. "Why Michelle Obama Chose Becoming as the Title of Her Upcoming Memoir," *Oprah.com*, November 12, 2018, https://www.oprah.com/oprahs bookclub/why-michelle-obama-chose-becoming-as-the-title-of-her-memoir.

9. Hanne Laceulle, *Aging and Self-Realization: Cultural Narratives about Later Life* (Germany: Transcript Verlag, 2018) 63–92.

10. Ada Calhoun, *Why We Can't Sleep, First Edition*. (New York: Grove Press, 2020), X.

11. Sara Scribner, "Generation X gets really old: How do slackers have a midlife crisis?," *Salon*, August 11, 2013, https://www.salon.com/2013/08/11/generation_x_gets_really_old_how_do_slackers_have_a_midlife_crisis.

12. James Gallagher, "Fertility rate: 'Jaw-dropping' global crash in children being born," *BBC*, July 15, 2020, https://www.bbc.com/news/health-53409521.

13. Renee Stepler, "Smaller Share of Women Ages 65 and Older Are Living Alone," *Pew Research Center*, February 18, 2016, https://www.pewsocialtrends.org/2016/02/18/smaller-share-of-women-ages-65-and-older-are-living-alone.

14. "Unmarried and Single Americans Week: Sept. 17–23, 2017," *US Census Bureau*, August 14, 2017, https://www.census.gov/newsroom/facts-for-features/2017/single-americans-week.html.

15. "Women More Likely Than Men to Initiate Divorces, But Not Non-Marital Breakups," *American Sociological Association*, August 22, 2015, https://www.asanet.org/press-center/press-releases/women-more-likely-men-initiate-divorces-not-non-marital-breakups.

16. Ann Marie Kerwin, "Cindy Gallop Doesn't Care What You Think, *Ad Age*, August 22, 2016, https://adage.com/article/news/cindi-gallop/305457.

17. "Ageism: The Last Acceptable Prejudice in America | Real Time with Bill Maher (HBO)," accessed March 23, 2021, https://www.youtube.com/watch?v=0kWaKhrpa28.

18. Alison Kafer, *Feminist, Queer, Crip* (Indiana University Press, 2013), 2.

19. Kafer, *Feminist, Queer, Crip*, 2.

CHAPTER 1

1. https://www.huffingtonpost.co.uk/mohadesa-najumi/ban-bossy-women-who-do-not-need-validation-are-feared_b_4971919.html.

2. https://www.imdb.com/title/tt3814440/characters/nm0000404.[

3. Lisa Anderson, "It's official: many women become invisible after 49," Thomson Reuters Foundation, accessed April 27, 2021, https://www.reuters.com/article/us-rights-women-ageing/its-official-many-women-become-invisible-after-49-idUSKBN0N41RH20150413.

4. Patricia Cohen, *In Our Prime: The Invention of Middle Age* (New York: Scribner, 2012), 40.

5. Cohen, *In Our Prime: The Invention of Middle Age*, 27.

6. Cohen, *In Our Prime: The Invention of Middle Age*, 28–29.

7. Cohen, *In Our Prime: The Invention of Middle Age*, 41.

8. Dr. David Reuben, *Everything You Ever Wanted to Know About Sex** (**But Were Afraid to Ask)*, (New York: McKay, 1969), 341.

9. "Everything You Always Wanted to Know About Sex* (*But Were Afraid to Ask)," The Woody Allen Pages, accessed April 27, 2021, http://www.woodyallenpages.com/films/everything-you-always-wanted-to-know-about-sex-but-were-afraid-to-ask.

10. S. J. Diamond, "Sequel / 'Phenomenon' Authors," *Los Angeles Times*, February 1, 1993, https://www.latimes.com/archives/la-xpm-1993-02-01-vw-992-story.html.

11. Alexandra Nikolchev, "A brief history of the birth control pill," PBS, accessed April 27, 2021, https://www.pbs.org/wnet/need-to-know/health/a-brief-history-of-the-birth-control-pill/480.

12. Martha Rampton, "Four Waves of Feminism," Pacific University Oregon, 2008, https://www.pacificu.edu/magazine/four-waves-feminism.

13. Dr. Jen Gunter, *The Menopause Manifesto: Own Your Health with Facts and Feminism* (New York: Citadel Press, 2021), X.

14. Francis Glennon, "Meaty Meadisms About America," *Life*, September 14, 1959, 47, No. 11, Google Books, accessed April 26, 2021, 147.

15. Susanne Schmidt, *Midlife Crisis: The Feminist Origins of a Chauvinist Cliché* (Chicago: University of Chicago Press, 2020), 20.

16. Schmidt, *Midlife Crisis*, 20.

17. Schmidt, *Midlife Crisis* 27.

18. Liza Mundy, "The Secret Power of Menopause," *The Atlantic*, accessed April 26, 2021, https://www.theatlantic.com/magazine/archive/2019/10/the-secret-power-of-menopause/596662.

19. Gunter, *The Menopause Manifesto: Own Your Health with Facts and Feminism*, X.

20. Marianne Hirsch, "Women's Ways of Aging," *Public Books*, June 16, 2020, https://www.publicbooks.org/womens-ways-of-aging.

21. Paula Span, "Aging Without Children," *New York Times*, March 25, 2011, https://newoldage.blogs.nytimes.com/2011/03/25/aging-without-children.

22. Michael J. Coren, "Are millennials really giving up on children over climate change?," *Quartz*, December 3, 2020, https://qz.com/1940690/are-millennials-really-giving-up-on-children-over-climate-change.

23. Dorthe Nors, "On the Invisibility of Middle-Aged Women," *Literary Hub*, June 22, 2016, https://lithub.com/on-the-invisibility-of-middle-aged-women.

24. U.S. Census Bureau, "Historical Marital Status Tables," December 2020, https://www.census.gov/data/tables/time-series/demo/families/marital.html.

25. Quoctrung Bui and Claire Cain Miller, "The Age That Women Have Babies: How a Gap Divides America," *New York Times*, August 4, 2018, https://www.nytimes.com/interactive/2018/08/04/upshot/up-birth-age-gap.html.

26. "Parenting in America," *Pew Research Center*, December 17, 2015, https://www.pewsocialtrends.org/2015/12/17/1-the-american-family-today.

27. Judy R. Strauss, "The Baby Boomers Meet Menopause: Fertility, Attractiveness, and Affective Response to the Menopausal Transition," *Sex Roles* 68 (2013): 77–90, https://doi.org/10.1007/s11199-011-0002-9.

28. Barbara Waxman, "Celebrate Life's Newest Stage: Middlescence," *Forbes*, August 29, 2016, https://www.forbes.com/sites/nextavenue/2016/08/29/celebrate-lifes-newest-stage-middlescence.

29. Swati Gupta and Sugam Pokharel, "Indian woman gives birth to twins at age of 73," *CNN*, September 6, 2019, https://www.cnn.com/2019/09/06/health/india-woman-73-gives-birth-scli-intl.

30. Kait Hanson, "New Hampshire woman gives birth at 57," *Today*, March 24, 2021, https://www.today.com/parents/new-hampshire-woman-gives-birth-57-t212902.

31. Richard Halstead, "Buck Institute in Novato expands reproduction research," *Marin Independent Journal*, September 30, 2019, https://www.marinij.com/2019/09/30/buck-institute-in-novato-expands-reproduction-research.

32. Shirley Chan, Alyssa Gomes, and Rama Shankar Singh, "Is menopause still evolving? Evidence from a longitudinal study of multiethnic populations and its relevance to women's health," *BMC Women's Health* 20, 74 (2020), https://doi.org/10.1186/s12905-020-00932-8.

33. Stacy L. Smith, Marc Choueiti, and Katherine Pieper, "Inclusion or Invisibility: Comprehensive Annenberg Report on Diversity in Entertainment," *Institute for Diversity and Empowerment at Annenberg*, February 22, 2016, https://annenberg.usc.edu/sites/default/files/2017/04/07/MDSCI_CARD_Report_FINAL_Exec_Summary.pdf.

34. "TENA partners with the Geena Davis Institute on Gender in Media to launch new 'Ageless Test' to tackle ageism in media," Geena Davis Institute on Gender in Media, October 19, 2020, https://seejane.org/gender-in-media-news-release/tena-partners-with-the-geena-davis-institute-on-gender-in-media-to-launch-new-ageless-test-to-tackle-ageism-in-media.

35. Jess Cartner-Morley, "Shades of 50: how the midlife woman went from invisible to the main event," *The Guardian*, March 21, 2020, https://www.theguardian.com/fashion/2020/mar/21/shades-of-50-how-the-midlife-woman-went-from-invisible-to-the-main-event.

36. Annie Karni, "Paulina Porizkova taking verbal 'shots,'" *New York Post*, October 17, 2010, https://nypost.com/2010/10/17/paulina-porizkova-taking-verbal-shots.

37. Cailley Chella, "Paulina Porizkova, 54, says she shares 'the truth' about being an older woman to help others: 'We are all in the same frickin' boat!,'" *The Daily Mail*, July 18, 2019, https://www.dailymail.co.uk/tvshowbiz/article-7263077/Paulina-Porizkova-54-says-shares-truth-older-woman-help-others.html.

38. Deborah Copaken, "The Case of the Vanishing Woman," Next Avenue, accessed April 27, 2021, https://www.nextavenue.org/case-vanishing -woman.

39. Jane Evans, The Uninvisibility Project, accessed June 2, 2021, https:// www.uninvisibility.com.

40. Jes Matsick, Mary Kruk, and Britney Wardecker. "Sexual Orientation, Femininity, and Attitudes Toward Menstruation Among Women: Implications for Menopause," *Innovation in Aging*, 4 (Suppl 1), (2020): 860, https:// doi.org/10.1093/geroni/igaa057.3173.

41. Monika Kehoe, "Lesbians over sixty-five: A triply invisible minority," *Journal of Homosexuality*, 12 (2020): 139–52, https://doi.org/10.1300/ J082v12n03_12.

42. Robert McRuer, *Crip Theory: Cultural Signs of Queerness and Disability* (New York: New York University Press, 2006.) 197.

43. "Disability Impacts All of Us," *Centers for Disease and Control*, September 16, 2020, https://www.cdc.gov/ncbddd/disabilityandhealth/infographic -disability-impacts-all.html.

44. Ola Ojewumi, "I'm Celebrating My Disabled Black Girl Magic Because I'm Done Feeling Invisible," *Self*, November 7, 2018, https://www.self .com/story/disabled-black-girl-magic.

45. Ola Ojewumi phone conversation, December 17, 2020.

46. Valerie Purdie-Vaughns and Richard P. Eibach, "Intersectional Invisibility: The Distinctive Advantages and Disadvantages of Multiple Subordinate-Group Identities," *Sex Roles* 59, (2008): 377–391, https://doi.org/10.1007/ s11199-008-9424-4.

47. "Dominant narratives on ageing," *Centre for Ageing Better*, November, 2020, https://www.ageing-better.org.uk/sites/default/files/2020-11/ dominant-narratives-ageing-full-report.pdf.

48. Aging Without Children Consultancy, February 25, 2021, https:// ageingwithoutchildrenconsultancy.com/2021/02/25/the-invisibility-of-peo ple-without-children-is-a-life-course-issue-which-has-a-drastic-impact-on -policy-around-age-and-ageing.

49. Kinneret Lahad, *A Table For One: A Critical Reading of Singlehood, Gender and Time* (England: Manchester University Press, 2017), 52.

50. McRuer, *Crip Theory*, 197.

51. Kathleen Schreurs, Anabel Quan-Haase, and Kim Martin. "Problematizing the Digital Literacy Paradox in the Context of Older Adults' ICT Use: Aging, Media Discourse, and Self-Determination," *Canadian Journal of Communication* 42.2 (2017): 359–77. Print.

52. Kandace L. Harris, "'Follow Me on Instagram': 'Best Self' Identity Construction and Gaze through Hashtag Activism and Selfie Self-Love," in *Women of Color and Social Media: Multitasking Blogs, Timelines, Feeds, and Community*, ed. S. M. Brown Givens and K. Edwards Tassie (Maryland: Lexington Books, 2015), 133.

53. Moya Bailey, *Misogynoir Transformed: Black Women's Digital Resistance* (New York: NYU Press 2021), X.
54. Laura McGrath, "Achieving Visibility: Midlife and Older Women's Literate Practices on Instagram and Blogs," *Literacy in Composition Studies,* 6 (2) (2018): https://licsjournal.org/index.php/LiCS/article/view/728.
55. Alessandra Bruni Lopez y Royo, "Modeling as an Older Woman: Exploitation or Subversion?," *Age Culture Humanities,* 2 (2015): 295–308, https://ageculturehumanities.org/WP/modeling-as-an-older-woman-ex ploitation-or-subversion.
56. "Sawubona: An African Tribe's Beautiful Greeting," *Exploring Your Mind,* October, 1, 2018, https://exploringyourmind.com/sawubona-african -tribe-greeting.
57. Akiko Busch, "The Invisibility of Older Women," *The Atlantic,* February 27, 2019, https://www.theatlantic.com/entertainment/archive/2019/02/ akiko-busch-mrs-dalloway-shows-aging-has-benefits/583480/.

CHAPTER 2

1. Erica Jong, *Fear of Dying* (New York: St. Martin's Griffin) 7–8.
2. Bianca Fileborn, et al., Sex, desire and pleasure: Considering the experiences of older Australian women. *Sexual and relationship therapy: Journal of the British Association for Sexual and Relationship Therapy,* 30 (1) (2015): 117–30, https://doi.org/10.1080/14681994.2014.936722.
3. Clare Kermond, "Older women want sex more, not less," *Sydney Morning Herald,* February 25, 2015, https://www.smh.com.au/lifestyle/life -and-relationships/older-women-want-sex-more-not-less-20150225-13oafi .html.
4. H. A. Feldman, et al., "Impotence and its medical and psychosocial correlates: Results of the Massachusetts Male Aging Study," *Journal of Urology* 151 (1994): 54–61, https://doi.org/10.1016/s0022-5347(17)34871-1.
5. Edward O. Laumann, A. Paik, R. C. Rosen, "Sexual dysfunction in the United States: Prevalence and predictors," *Journal of the American Medical Association* 281 (6) (1999): 537–44, https://doi.org/10.1001/jama.281.6.537.
6. Bruce Lee, "Can Covid-19 Coronavirus Cause Long-Term Erectile Dysfunction? Here Are 2 More Studies," *Forbes,* May 16, 2021, https://www .forbes.com/sites/brucelee/2021/05/16/can-covid-19-coronavirus-cause -long-term-erectile-dysfunction-here-are-2-more-studies.
7. Sarah Hunter Murray, "Heterosexual Men's Sexual Desire: Supported by, or Deviating from, Traditional Masculinity Norms and Sexual Scripts?" *Sex Roles* 78 (2018): 130–41, https://doi.org/10.1007/s11199-017-0766-7.
8. Michelle Maciel and Luciana Laganà, "Older women's sexual desire problems: Biopsychosocial factors impacting them and barriers to their

clinical assessment," *BioMed research international,* 107–217, (2014), https://doi.org/10.1155/2014/107217.

9. Denise Petski, "Emma Thompson Criticizes the "Utterly Unbalanced" Casting of Older Men With Much Younger Women," *Deadline,* December 25, 2020, https://deadline.com/2020/12/emma-thompson-criticizes-the-utterly-unbalanced-casting-of-older-men-with-much-younger-women-1234661562.

10. Hayley Stainton, "Female sex tourism. What does it mean and where does it happen?" Tourism Teacher, accessed Jan 6, 2021, https://tourismteacher.com/female-sex-tourism.

11. Aurora Snow, "Career-Minded Women Turn to Male Escorts for No-Strings Fun and (Maybe) Sex," *The Daily Beast,* January 3, 2015, https://www.thedailybeast.com/career-minded-women-turn-to-male-escorts-for-no-strings-fun-and-maybe-sex?

12. Hilary Caldwell and John de Wit, "Women's experiences buying sex in Australia—Egalitarian power moves," *Sexualities* 24, no. 4 (June 2021): 549–73, https://doi.org/10.1177/1363460719896972.

13. David A. Frederick, et al., "Differences in Orgasm Frequency Among Gay, Lesbian, Bisexual, and Heterosexual Men and Women in a U.S. National Sample," *Archives of sexual behavior,* 47 (1) (2018): 273–88, https://doi.org/10.1007/s10508-017-0939-z.

14. Linda Kirkman, "Relationship diversity and the life span: Rural baby boomers in friend-with-benefits relationships," paper presented at the Let's Talk About Sex Conference, Pullman on the Park, Melbourne, Victoria, Australia (September 9, 2015).

15. Cindy Gallop phone call, January 25, 2020.

16. "The Case For An Older Woman," OkCupid, February 16, 2010, https://theblog.okcupid.com/the-case-for-an-older-woman-99d8cabacdf5.

17. "For women, sexuality changes with age but doesn't disappear," Harvard Health Publishing, July 21, 2019, https://www.health.harvard.edu/blog/for-women-sexuality-changes-with-age-but-doesnt-disappear-201402137035.

18. Judy G. Bretschneider and Norma L. McCoy, "Sexual interest and behavior in healthy 80- to 102-year-olds," *Archives of Sexual Behavior* 17 (1988): 109–29, https://doi.org/10.1007/BF01542662.

19. Cynthia A. Graham, et al., "What factors are associated with reporting lacking interest in sex and how do these vary by gender? Findings from the third British national survey of sexual attitudes and lifestyles," British Medical Journal Open vol. 7, 9 e016942 (September 13, 2017), doi:10.1136/bmjopen-2017-016942.

20. Emily Allen Paine, Debra Umberson, and Corinne Reczek, "Sex in Midlife: Women's Sexual Experiences in Lesbian and Straight Marriages," *Journal of marriage and the family, 81* (1) (2019): 7–23, https://doi.org/10.1111/jomf.12508.

21. Alina Kao et al, "Dyspareunia in postmenopausal women: A critical review," *Pain research & management, 13* (3) (2008): 243–54, https://doi.org/10.1155/2008/269571.

22. Sheryl A. Kingsberg and Terri Woodard, "Female sexual dysfunction: Focus on low desire," *Obstetrics and gynecology*, 125(2) (2015): 477–86, https://doi.org/10.1097/AOG.0000000000000620.

23. M. J. Kaas, "Geriatric sexuality breakdown syndrome," *The International Journal of Aging and Human Development*, 13 (1) (1981): 71–77, https://doi.org/10.2190/4A16-06AH-HL5A-WKC3.

24. Margaret A. Salisu and Jagadisa-Devasri Dacus, "Living in a Paradox: How Older Single and Widowed Black Women Understand Their Sexuality," *Journal of Gerontological Social Work*, 64:3 (2021): 303–33, https://doi.*org*/10.1080/01634372.2020.1870603

25. Salisu and Dacus, "Living in a Paradox: How Older Single and Widowed Black Women Understand Their Sexuality," 303–33.

26. Luciana Laganá, et al., "Exploring the Sexuality of African American Older Women," *British journal of medicine and medical research*, 4(5), (2013): 1129–48, https://doi.org/10.9734/BJMMR/2014/5491.

27. Liza Berdychevsky and Galit Nimrod, "Sex as Leisure in Later life: A Netnographic Approach," *Leisure Sciences*, 39:3 (2017): 224–43, http://dx.doi.org/10.1080/01490400.2016.1189368.

28. "Singles in America: Match Releases Largest Study on U.S. Single Population for Eighth Year," accessed May 15, 2021, https://www.prnewswire.com/news-releases/singles-in-america-match-releases-largest-study-on-us-single-population-for-eighth-year-300591561.html.

29. Wednesday Martin, *Untrue: Why Nearly Everything We Believe About Women, Lust, and Infidelity Is Wrong and How the New Science Can Set Us Free* (New York: Little, Brown Spark, 2018), 42.

30. Esther Perel, *The State of Affairs: Rethinking Infidelity* (New York: Harper, 2017), 185.

31. Barbara J. Risman, Carissa Froyum, and William Scarborough, editors. *Handbook on the Sociology of Gender* (New York: Springer Publishers, 2018).

32. Maciel and Laganà, "Older women's sexual desire problems: Biopsychosocial factors impacting them and barriers to their clinical assessment (2014).

33. Berdychevsky and Nimrod, "Sex as Leisure in Later life: A Netnographic Approach," 224–43.

34. Robin Wilson-Beattie, "Bodies in Transition," *Pulp*, December 10, 2019, https://medium.com/pulpmag/bodies-in-transition-34020653f782.

35. Emma McGowan, "The Sex Educator Teaching BDSM to People With Disabilities," *Vice*, December, 4, 2017, https://www.vice.com/en/article/ywnm7v/robin-wilson-beattie-sex-educator-bdsm-disabilities?.

36. Alexandra H. Solomon phone call, March 8, 2021.

37. Lorraine Dennerstein, Ph.D, Philippe Lehert, Ph.D., Henry Burger, M.D., "The relative effects of hormones and relationship factors on sexual

function of women through the natural menopausal transition," *Reproductive endocrinology* 84, 1 (2005): 174–80, https://doi.org/10.1016/j.fertn stert.2005.01.119.

38. Kate A. Morrissey Stahl, et al., "Sex after divorce: Older adult women's reflections," *Journal of Gerontological Social Work*, 61(6) (2018): 659–74, https://doi.org/10.1080/01634372.2018.1486936.

39. Nicole Brodeur, "'Love and Trouble': Claire Dederer's midlife take on sex and self-perception," *The Seattle Times*, May 5, 2021, https://www.seattletimes.com/entertainment/books/why-was-i-a-gigantic-slut-claire-dederers-midlife-take-on-love-sex-and-trouble.

40. Ada Calhoun, *Wedding Toasts I'll Never Give* (New York: W. W. Norton Company, 2017), 44.

41. Kim Brooks, "The Emancipation of the MILF," *The Cut*, May 18, 2017, https://www.thecut.com/2017/05/female-sexuality-desire-what-happens-as-women-age.html.

42. Kim Brooks, "Married With Benefits," *Chicago Magazine*, April, 23, 2019, https://www.chicagomag.com/Chicago-Magazine/May-2019/Married-With-Benefits.

43. Kim Brooks and The Cut, "The changing reasons why women cheat on their husbands," *CNN*, March 13, 2018, https://www.cnn.com/2017/10/05/health/why-women-cheat-partner/index.html.

44. Perel, *The State of Affairs: Rethinking Infidelity*, 183.

45. J. D. Drummond, et al., "The impact of caregiving: Older women's experiences of sexuality and intimacy," *Affilia: Journal of Women & Social Work*, 28(4) (2013): 415–28, https://doi.org/10.1177/0886109913504154.

46. Cheryl Brown Travis and C. P. Yeager, "Sexual Selection, Parental Investment, and Sexism," *Journal of Social Issues*, 47 (1991): 117–29, https://doi.org/10.1111/j.1540-4560.1991.tb01826.x.

47. Ali Ziegler, et al., "Does monogamy harm women? Deconstructing monogamy with a feminist lens," [Special Issue on Polyamory]. *Journal für Psychologie*, 22(1) (2014): 1–18, https://www.journal-fuer-psychologie.de/index.php/jfp/article/view/323/354.

48. David C. Atkins, Donald H. Baucom, and Neil S. Jacobson, "Understanding infidelity: Correlates in a national random sample," *Journal of Family Psychology*, 15(4) (2001): 735–49, https://doi.org/10.1037/0893-3200.15.4.735.

49. Jill Bialosky, "How We Became Strangers" in *The Bitch in the House: 26 Women Tell the Truth About Sex, Solitude, Work, Motherhood, and Marriage*, ed. Cathi Hanauer (New York: William Morrow Paperbacks, 2003), 119.

50. Alice Walker, *Secret Life of the Cheating Wife: Power, Pragmatism, and Pleasure in Women's Infidelity* (Maryland: Lexington Books, 2017) 131–32.

51. Kim Brooks, "Why So Many Women Cheat on Their Husbands, *The Cut*, September 21, 2017, https://www.thecut.com/2017/09/why-women-cheat-esther-perel-state-of-affairs.html.

52. Tessa and Amir, The Open Nesters, personal phone call, January 2021.

53. Elle Beau, "Hot Sex Is Not Just for the Young," *Sensual: An Erotic Life*, December 13, 2020, https://medium.com/sensual-enchantment/hot-sex is -not-just-for-the-young-fc2ffcec93ba.

54. Elle Beau, "Hot Sex Is Not Just for the Young."

55. Elizabeth Gilbert, *Facebook*, July 1, 2016.

56. Kristin Tillotson, "Many Women Come Out as Lesbians Later in Life, *Star Tribune* (Minneapolis), January 21, 2010, https://www.post andcourier.com/features/many-women-come-out-as-lesbians-later-in-life/article_6be6af57-e9ee-5f44-a4bc-9b17dba0ed59.html.

57. Nancy C. Larson, "Becoming 'One of the Girls: The Transition to Lesbian in Midlife,'" *Affilia*, 21 (2006): 296–305, https://doi.org/10.1177/0886109906288911.

58. Kira Cochrane, "Why it's never too late to be a lesbian," *The Guardian*, July 22, 2010, https://www.theguardian.com/lifeandstyle/2010/jul/22/late -blooming-lesbians-women-sexuality.

59. Anna Moore. "The sexuality revolution: 'Switching sides' in midlife," *You magazine*, July 15, 2018, https://www.you.co.uk/changing-sexuality-in -midlife/.

60. Paige Averett., Intae Yoon, and Carol L. Jenkins. Older lesbian sexuality: Identity, sexual behavior, and the impact of aging. *Journal of sex research*, 49(5) (2012): 495–507, https://doi.org/10.1080/00224499.2011.582543.

61. Martha B. Holstein, PhD and Meredith Minkler, Dr. PH, "Self, Society, and the 'New Gerontology,'" *The Gerontologist*, Vol. 43, Issue 6 (December 2003): 787–96, https://doi.org/10.1093/geront/43.6.787.

62. Stephen Katz and Barbara Marshall, "New sex for old: Lifestyle, consumerism, and the ethics of aging well," *Journal of Aging Studies*, 17 (2003): 3–16, https://doi.org/10.1016/S0890-4065(02)00086-5.

63. Dr. Jen Gunter, "When the Cause of a Sexless Relationship Is—Surprise!—the Man," *New York Times*, March 10, 2018, https://www.nytimes.com/2018/03/10/style/sexless-relationships-men-low-libido.html.

64. Sharron Hinchliff, "When it comes to older people and sex, doctors put their heads in the sand," *The Conversation*, June 19, 2015, https://theconversation.com/when-it-comes-to-older-people-and-sex-doctors-put-their -heads-in-the-sand-43556.

65. Luciana Lagana and Michelle Maciel, "Sexual desire among Mexican-American older women: A qualitative study," *Culture, Health & Sexuality*, 6 (2010): 705–19, https://doi.org/10.1080/13691058.2010.482673.

66. Robin Wilson-Beattie, "Bodies in Transition."

67. Sandee LaMotte, "It's a myth that women don't want sex as they age, study finds," *CNN*, September 28, 2020, https://www.cnn.com/2020/09/28/health/sexual-desire-older-women-study-wellness/index.html.

CHAPTER 3

1. Paris Lees, "Emma Watson on Being Happily 'Self-Partnered' at 30," *Vogue*, April 15, 2020, https://www.vogue.co.uk/news/article/emma-watson-on-fame-activism-little-women.

2. Elizabeth Brake, *Minimizing Marriage: Marriage, Morality, and the Law* (England: Oxford University Press, 2012), 5.

3. Megan Garber, "When *Newsweek* 'Struck Terror in the Hearts of Single Women,'" *The Atlantic*, June 2016, https://www.theatlantic.com/entertainment/archive/2016/06/more-likely-to-be-killed-by-a-terrorist-than-to-get-married/485171.

4. U.S. Census Bureau, "Number, Timing, and Duration of Marriages and Divorces: 2009," May 2011, https://www.census.gov/prod/2011pubs/p70-125.pdf.

5. Deborah van den Hoonaard, "Attitudes of older widows and widowers in New Brunswick, Canada toward new partnerships," *Ageing International*, 27, 4 (2002): 79–92, https://doi.org/10.1007/s12126-002-1016-y.

6. Regina Kenen, "Suddenly Single: A Widow's Challenge," *The Society Pages*, July 5, 2018 https://thesocietypages.org/specials/suddenly-single-a-widows-challenge/.

7. "Settling for less out of fear of being single," Correction to Spielmann et al., *Journal of personality and social psychology*, 115(5) (2013) (2018): 804, https://doi.org/10.1037/pspp0000227.

8. Tierney McAfee, "Antonin Scalia Was with Members of Secretive Society of Elite Hunters When He Died," *People*, February 25, 2016, https://people.com/sports/antonin-scalia-died-during-getaway-with-members-of-secret-hunting-society.

9. Holly Nelson-Becker and Christina Victor, "Dying alone and lonely dying: Media discourse and pandemic conditions," *Journal of aging studies*, 55, 100878 (2020), https://doi.org/10.1016/j.jaging.2020.100878.

10. Anke C. Plagnol and Richard A. Easterlin, "Aspirations, Attainments, and Satisfaction: Life Cycle Differences Between American Women and Men," *Journal of Happiness Studies* 9 (2008): 601–19, https://doi.org/10.1007/s10902-008-9106-5.

11. Vanessa Fabbre, "Gender Transitions in Later Life: The Significance of Time in Queer Aging," *Journal of Gerontological Social Work*, 57(2–4) (2014): 161–75, https://doi.org/10.1080/01634372.2013.855287.

12. Institute of Medicine (US) Committee on Lesbian, Gay, Bisexual, and Transgender Health Issues and Research Gaps and Opportunities, "Later Adulthood," in *The Health of Lesbian, Gay, Bisexual, and Transgender People: Building a Foundation for Better Understanding* (Washington, DC: National Academies Press; 2011), https://www.ncbi.nlm.nih.gov/books/NBK64800.

13. Vicki Larson, "Marin psychotherapist addresses marriage at midlife in new book," *Marin Independent Journal*, January 22, 2018, https://www

.marinij.com/2018/01/22/marin-psychotherapist-addresses-marriage-at
-midlife-in-new-book.

14. Vicki Larson, "You can't avoid divorce, and here's why," *OMG Chronicles*, July 28, 2014, http://omgchronicles.vickilarson.com/2014/07/28/you-cant-avoid-divorce-and-heres-why.

15. Susan L. Brown and I-Fen Lin, "The Gray Divorce Revolution: Rising Divorce Among Middle-Aged and Older Adults, 1990–2010," *The Journals of Gerontology: Series B*, Vol. 67, Issue 6 (November 2012): 731–41, https://doi.org/10.1093/geronb/gbs089.

16. Renee Stepler, "Led by Baby Boomers, divorce rates climb for America's 50+ population," *Pew Research Center*, March 9, 2017, https://www.pewresearch.org/fact-tank/2017/03/09/led-by-baby-boomers-divorce-rates-climb-for-americas-50-population.

17. Paula England and Elizabeth Aura McClintock, "The Gendered Double Standard of Aging in US Marriage Markets," *Population and Development Review* 35(4) (2009): 797–816, https://doi.org/10.1111/j.1728-4457.2009.00309.x.

18. American Sociological Association, "Women more likely than men to initiate divorces, but not non-marital breakups," *ScienceDaily*, www.sciencedaily.com/releases/2015/08/150822154900.htm; Margaret F. Brinig and Douglas W. Allen, "'These boots are made for walking': Why most divorce filers are women," *American Law and Economics Review*, Volume 2, Issue 1, (January 2000): 126–69, https://doi.org/10.1093/aler/2.1.126.

19. Misty L. Heggeness, "The Up Side of Divorce?: When Laws Make Divorce Easier, Research Shows Women Benefit, Outcomes Improve," *U.S. Census Bureau*, https://www.census.gov/library/stories/2019/12/the-upside-of-divorce.html.

20. Jocelyn Elise Crowley, "Baby boomers are divorcing for surprisingly old-fashioned reasons," *Aeon*, May 7, 2018, https://aeon.co/ideas/baby-boomers-are-divorcing-for-surprisingly-old-fashioned-reasons.

21. Maya Luetke and others, "Romantic Relationship Conflict Due to the COVID-19 Pandemic and Changes in Intimate and Sexual Behaviors in a Nationally Representative Sample of American Adults," *Journal of Sex & Marital Therapy*, 46:8 (2020) 747–62, https://doi.org/10.1080/0092623X.2020.1810185.

22. Robert H. Coombs, "Marital Status and Personal Well-Being: A Literature Review," *Family Relations* 40, no. 1 (1991): 97–102. https://doi.org/10.2307/585665.

23. Lisa Wade, "Women are less happy than men in marriage, so why does the media insist otherwise?," *Sociological Images*, December 27, 2016, https://thesocietypages.org/socimages/2016/12/27/women-are-less-happy-than-men-in-marriage-so-why-does-the-media-insist-otherwise.

24. Tristan Bridges and Melody L. Boyd, "On Straight Men's Marriageability Across the Class Divide," *Feminist Reflections*, December 7,

2016, https://thesocietypages.org/feminist/2016/12/07/on-straight-mens-marriageability-across-the-class-divide.

25. Stephanie Coontz, "How to Make Your Marriage Gayer," *New York Times*, February 13, 2020, https://www.nytimes.com/2020/02/13/opinion/sunday/marriage-housework-gender-happiness.html.

26. Cynthia Grant Bowman, "Living Apart Together as a 'Family Form' Among Persons of Retirement Age: The Appropriate Family Law Response," *Family Law Quarterly* 52, 1 (2018): 1–25.

27. Zosia Bielski, "The new reality of dating over 65: Men want to live together; women don't," *The Globe and Mail*, November 26, 2019, https://www.theglobeandmail.com/life/relationships/article-women-older-than-65-dont-want-to-live-with-their-partners.

28. Diane Burke email March 12, 2021.

29. Isabelle Tessier, "I Want To Be Single—But With You," *Huff-Post*, July 17, 2015, https://www.huffpost.com/entry/i-to-be-single-but-with-you_b_7818158.

30. Bowman, "Living Apart Together as a 'Family Form' Among Persons of Retirement Age: The Appropriate Family Law Response."

31. Minda Zetlin, "Will Staying Home Lead to More Divorces? 45 Percent of Millennials and Gen-Z Say Yes," *Inc.*, April 17, 2020, https://www.inc.com/minda-zetlin/divorce-rates-coronavirus-relationships-strain-social-distancing.html.

32. "Singing spinster strikes a chord," *Associated Press*, April 17, 2009, https://www.dailynews.com/2009/04/17/singing-spinster-strikes-a-chord.

33. Rick Fulton, "Susan Boyle's life story to be turned into movie with Meryl Streep," *Daily Record*, November 21, 2019, https://www.dailyrecord.co.uk/news/scottish-news/movie-scots-superstar-susan-boyles-20925022.

34. Nicole Pasulka, "'Cat Knows How to Ignore Men': A Brief History of Lesbian Cat Ladies," *The Cut*, June 23, 2016, https://www.thecut.com/2016/06/brief-history-of-lesbian-cat-ladies.html.

35. Emerald Pellot, "Meet Astala Vista, the self-proclaimed 'crazy cat lady of drag,'" *In the Know*, January 25, 2021, https://www.intheknow.com/post/meet-astala-vista-the-self-proclaimed-crazy-cat-lady-of-drag.

36. Irene Reti and Shoney Sien, editors, *Cats (and their Dykes): An Anthology* (California: HerBooks, 1991), X.

37. Karin Lövgren, "The Swedish *tant*: A marker of female aging." *Journal of women & aging*, 25(2) (2013): 119–37, https://doi.org/10.1080/08952841.2013.732826.

38. Katie Sullivan Barak, "Spinsters, old maids, and cat ladies: A case study in containment strategies" (PhD diss., Bowling Green State University, 2014), 1–221, https://etd.ohiolink.edu/apexprod/rws_etd/send_file/send?accession=bgsu1393246792&disposition=inline.

39. Rob Picheta, "'Crazy cat ladies' are not a thing, study finds," *CNN*, August 21, 2019, https://www.cnn.com/2019/08/21/health/crazy-cat-lady-study-scli-intl/index.html.

40. Trish Hafford-Letchfield and others, "Going Solo: Findings from a survey of women ageing without a partner and who do not have children," *Journal of Women & Aging* Vol. 29,4 (2017): 321–33, doi:10.1080/08952841.20 16.1187544.

41. I-Fen Lin, PhD and Susan L. Brown, PhD, "Unmarried Boomers Confront Old Age: A National Portrait," *The Gerontologist,* Volume 52, Issue 2 (April 2012): 153–65, https://doi.org/10.1093/geront/gnr141.

42. "Relationship Status: Single—Dating Perceptions and Behaviors Among Generation X and Boomers," *AARP,* February 2019, https://doi.org/10.26419/res.00278.004.

43. "Aging baby boomers, childless and unmarried, at risk of becoming 'elder orphans,'" *Eureka Alert,* May 15, 2015, https://www.eurekalert.org/pub_releases/2015-05/nsij-abb051315.php.

44. Katie Bindley, "Gen X Women Succeed at Work, Have Fewer Kids: Study," *HuffPost,* September 13, 2011, https://www.huffpost.com/entry/gen-x-study_n_959256.

45. Brady E. Hamilton, Ph.D., Joyce A. Martin, M. P. H., and Michelle J. K. Osterman, M.H.S., "Births: Provisional Data for 2019," Division of Vital Statistics, National Center for Health Statistics, May 2020, https://www.cdc.gov/nchs/data/vsrr/vsrr-8-508.pdf.

46. Zhenmei Zhang and Mark D. Hayward, "Childlessness and the Psychological Well-Being of Older Persons," *The Journals of Gerontology: Series B,* 56, Issue 5, 1 (September 2001): S311–S320, https://doi.org/10.1093/geronb/56.5.S311; Małgorzata Mikucka, "Old-Age Trajectories of Life Satisfaction. Do Singlehood and Childlessness Hurt More When People Get Older?," *Swiss Journal of Sociology* 46, 3 (2020): 397–424, doi: https://doi.org/10.2478/sjs-2020-0020.

47. Trish Hafford-Letchfield and others "Going Solo: Findings from a survey of women ageing without a partner and who do not have children"; Eileen Reilly, Trish Hafford-Letchfield, and Nicky Lambert, "Women ageing solo in Ireland: An exploratory study of women's perspectives on relationship status and future care needs," *Qualitative Social Work,* 19(1) (August 28, 2018): 75–92, https://doi.org/10.1177/1473325018796138.

48. Rudly Raphael, "What Women Want: Love, Marriage and Dating," *Ebony,* March 7, 2019, https://www.ebony.com/life/ebony-attitudes/what-women-want-love-marriage-and-dating.

49. Apryl Motley, "Single and Loving It," *Sisters from AARP,* November 15, 2019, https://www.sistersletter.com/me-time/single-and-loving-it.

50. Institute on Aging, https://www.ioaging.org/aging-in-america.

51. Joshua Coleman, "A Shift in American Family Values," *The Atlantic,* January 10, 2021, https://www.theatlantic.com/family/archive/2021/01/why-parents-and-kids-get-estranged/617612.

52. Jody Day, "I'm Losing My Shame," *The Age Buster,* November 20, 2020, https://www.theagebuster.com/blog-page/2020/11/20/im-losing-my-shame.

53. Rich Benjamin, "Op-Ed: The president-elect and his VP both provide great models for matrimony," *Los Angeles Times*, November 15, 2020, https://www.latimes.com/opinion/story/2020-11-15/the-president-elect-and-his-veep.

54. Rachel DeSantis and Charlotte Triggs, "Sheryl Sandberg Is Engaged to Tom Bernthal After Being Set Up by Her Late Husband's Brother," *People*, February 3, 2020, https://people.com/human-interest/sheryl-sandberg-engaged-tom-bernthal.

55. Lois Smith Brady, "The Writer Anne Lamott Gets to the Happily-Ever-After Part," *New York Times*, April 26, 2019, https://www.nytimes.com/2019/04/26/fashion/weddings/the-final-chapters-of-anne-lamotts-life-now-include-a-soul-mate.html.

56. Paula England and Elizabeth Aura McClintock, "The Gendered Double Standard of Aging in US Marriage Markets," *Population and Development Review, The Population Council, Inc.*, 35(4) (December 2009): 797–816.

57. "Relationship Status: Single—Dating Perceptions and Behaviors Among Generation X and Boomers," *AARP*.

58. Wendy K. Watson and Charlie Stelle, "Dating for older women: Experiences and meanings of dating in later life," *Journal of Women & Aging*, 23(3) (2011): 263–75, https://doi.org/10.1080/08952841.2011.587732.

59. Gina Potârcă, Melinda Mills, and Wiebke Neberich "Relationship Preferences Among Gay and Lesbian Online Daters: Individual and Contextual Influences," *Journal of Marriage and Family*, 77(2) (2015): 523–41, https://doi.org/10.1111/jomf.12177.

60. Michael J. Rosenfeld, "Who Wants the Breakup? Gender and Breakup in Heterosexual Couples," in *Social Networks and the Life Course: Integrating the Development of Human Lives and Social Relational Networks*, First Edition, ed. Duane F. Alwin, Diane Felmlee, and Derek Kreager (New York: Springer, 2018), 221–43.

61. Faith Hill, "What It's Like to Date After Middle Age," *The Atlantic*, January 8, 2020, https://www.theatlantic.com/family/archive/2020/01/dating-after-middle-age-older/604588/.

62. Gail Sheehy, *Sex and the Seasoned Woman: Pursuing the Passionate Life* (New York: Ballantine Books, 2007), 53.

63. Vicki Larson, "Never too late to find love, says Mill Valley's Eve Pell," *The Marin Independent Journal*, January 26, 2015, https://www.marinij.com/2015/01/26/never-too-late-to-find-love-says-mill-valleys-eve-pell.

64. Philip Cohen, "Marriage rates among people with disabilities (save the data edition)," *The Society Pages*, November 11, 2014, https://thesocietypages.org/ccf/2014/11/24/marriage-rates-among-people-with-disabilities-save-the-data-edition.

65. Emma McGowan, "The Sex Educator Teaching BDSM to People With Disabilities."

66. Kelly Raley, Megan M. Sweeney, and Danielle Wondra, "The Growing Racial and Ethnic Divide in U.S. Marriage Patterns," *The Future of Children*, 25(2) (2015): 89–109, https://doi.org/10.1353/foc.2015.0014.

67. Nicole Cardos, "Why One Sociologist Says It's Time for Black Women to Date White Men," WTTW, April 17, 2019, https://news.wttw.com/2019/04/17/sociologist-cheryl-judice-interracial-relationships.

68. Paige Averett phone call, February 12, 2021.

69. Michael J. Rosenfeld, "Are Tinder and Dating Apps Changing Dating and Mating in the U.S.?" in *Families and Technology*, ed. Jennifer Van Hook, Susan M. McHale, and Valarie King (New York: Springer, 2018). 103–17.

70. Michael J. Rosenfeld and Reuben J. Thomas, "Searching for a Mate: The Rise of the Internet as a Social Intermediary," *American Sociological Review*, 77 (2012): 523–47, https://doi.org/10.1177/0003122412448050.

71. Rebecca P. Yu and others, "Mapping the Two Levels of Digital Divide: Internet Access and Social Network Site Adoption among Older Adults in the USA," *Information, Communication & Society*, 19, 10 (2016): 1445–64, https://doi.org/10.1080/1369118X.2015.1109695.

72. Ahro Ko and others, "Family Matters: Rethinking the Psychology of Human Social Motivation," *Perspectives on Psychological Science* 15, no. 1 (January 2020): 173–201, https://doi.org/10.1177/1745691619872986.

CHAPTER 4

1. Tracy Letts, *August: Osage County* (page 51).

2. https://www.marieclaire.fr/yann-moix-rompre-interview,1291590.asp.

3. Amanda Cundall and Kun Guo, "Women gaze behaviour in assessing female bodies: The effects of clothing, body size, own body composition and body satisfaction," *Psychological Research* 81 (2017): 1–12, https://doi.org/10.1007/s00426-015-0726-1.

4. Alexandra H. Solomon, *Taking Sexy Back: How to Own Your Sexuality and Create the Relationships You Want* (California: New Harbinger Publications, 2019), 104.

5. Colette Thayer, "Mirror/Mirror: AARP Survey of Women's Reflections on Beauty, Age, and Media," *AARP Research* (October 2018), https://doi.org/10.26419/res.00250.001.

6. Anne E. Barrett and Cheryl Robbins, "The Multiple Sources of Women's Aging Anxiety and Their Relationship With Psychological Distress," *Journal of Aging & Health*, 20 (1) (2008): 32–65, https://doi.org/10.1177/0898264307309932.

7. Holly N. Thomas and others, "Body Image, Attractiveness, and Sexual Satisfaction Among Midlife Women: A Qualitative Study," *Journal of Women's Health* 28, 1 (2002): 100–106. https://doi.org/10.1089/jwh.2018.7107.

8. Barrett and Robbins, "The Multiple Sources of Women's Aging Anxiety and Their Relationship With Psychological Distress."

9. Renee Engeln, *Beauty Sick: How the Cultural Obsession with Appearance Hurts Girls and Women* (New York: HarperCollins Publishers, 2017) 7–8.

10. Katie Kilkenny, "How Anti-Aging Cosmetics Took Over the Beauty World," *Pacific Standard,* August 30, 2017, https://psmag.com/social-justice/how-anti-aging-cosmetics-took-over-the-beauty-world.

11. Cheryl Wischhover, "The fall of "anti-aging" skin care," *Vox,* September 11, 2018, https://www.vox.com/the-goods/2018/9/11/17840984/skin-care-anti-aging-drunk-elephant.

12. Amarendra Pandey, Gurpoonam K. Jatana and Sidharth Sonthalia, "Cosmeceuticals," in *StatPearls* (Florida: StatPearls Publishing, 2020), https://www.ncbi.nlm.nih.gov/books/NBK544223.

13. Krista Bennett DeMaio and Erin Stovall, "Beauty Brands Are Catering to Women Over 50—Finally," *Oprah Daily,* February 19, 2020, https://www.oprahmag.com/beauty/a30980789/beauty-brands-women-over-50/.

14. "That Age Old Question: How Attitudes to Ageing Affect Our Health and Wellbeing," *Royal Society for Public Health,* May 10, 2018, https://www.rsph.org.uk/static/uploaded/a01e3aa7-9356-40bc-99c81b14dd904a41.pdf.

15. Jennifer Lopez @jlo, Instagram, January 15, 2021, https://www.instagram.com/tv/CKFecOZpEeL/?hl=en.

16. American Society of Plastic Surgeons, "2018 Plastic Surgery Statistics Report," https://www.plasticsurgery.org/documents/News/Statistics/2018/plastic-surgery-statistics-full-report-2018.pdf.

17. Rebecca M. Herzig, *Plucked: A History of Hair Removal* (New York: New York University Press, 2015), 17.

18. Justine Bateman, *Face: One Square Foot of Skin* (New York: Akashic, 2021), 14.

19. Annette Bening, "Acting Is 'A Fabulous Way To Expand Your Own Heart,'" interview by Terry Gross, *Fresh Air,* NPR, May 10, 2018, audio, 36:00, http://www.npr. /2018/05/10/610014961/annette-bening-acting-is-a-fabulous-way-to-expand-your-own-heart.

20. Clare Mehta, "At what age are people usually happiest? New research offers surprising clues," *The Conversation,* April 9, 2021, https://theconversation.com/at-what-age-are-people-usually-happiest-new-research-offers-surprising-clues-156906.

21. Tim Appelo, "Geena Davis Calls Hollywood's Age Bias 'Dismal,'" *AARP,* November 4, 2020, https://www.aarp.org/entertainment/movies-for-grownups/info-2020/geena-davis-actresses-ageism-in-hollywood.html.

22. Frances McDormand, "Like Olive Kitteridge, Actress Frances McDormand Was Tired of Supporting Roles," interview by Melissa Block, *All Things Considered,* NPR, October 31, 2014, audio, 8:00, https://www.npr.org/2014/10/31/360183633/like-olive-kitteridge-actress-frances-mcdormand-was-tired-of-supporting-roles.

23. Paul Liberatore, "Frances McDormand, Marin's media-shy star, lends support to coastal radio station," *Marin Independent Journal*, December 15, 2014, https://www.marinij.com/2014/12/15/frances-mcdormand-marins-media-shy-star-lends-support-to-coastal-radio-station.

24. Pandora Amoratis, "Go au naturale! From letting nails breathe to air drying hair like Ariana Grande, beauty experts reveal why it's a good idea to embrace the natural look while in quarantine," *The Daily Mail*, April 16, 2020, https://www.dailymail.co.uk/femail/article-8221941/Beauty-experts-reveal-look-better-later.html.

25. Manoush Zomorodi, "A Self-Indulgent Ode to Old Lady Hair," *Human Parts*, November 17, 2020, https://humanparts.medium.com/old-lady-hair-a67eb312ae8c.

26. Cristine Russell, "Hair Today, Gray Tomorrow," *Washington Post*, October 8, 1989, https://www.washingtonpost.com/archive/lifestyle/wellness/1989/10/08/hair-today-gray-tomorrow/7abc2f13-e8b7-4f9b-a1d8-08a88cc15668.

27. Ségolène Panhard, Isabelle Lozano, and Geneviève Loussouarn, "Greying of the human hair: A worldwide survey, revisiting the '50' rule of thumb," *The British Journal of Dermatology*, 167, 4 (2012): 865–73, https://doi.org/10.1111/j.1365-2133.2012.11095.x.

28. Deanna Pai, "The Gray-Hair Revolution Has Begun," *Glamour*, January 29, 2019, https://www.glamour.com/story/gray-hair-revolution.

29. Clayton Edwards, "'The Golden Girls': Who Was the Youngest Actress on the Show?," *Outsider*, April 1, 2021, https://outsider.com/news/entertainment/golden-girls-who-was-youngest-actress-on-show.

30. Justine Coupland and Richard Gwyn, editors, *Discourse, the Body, and Identity* (New York, Palgrave Macmillan, 2003), 128.

31. Sonya Renee Taylor, *The Body Is Not an Apology Second Edition: The Power of Radical Self-Love* (California: Berrett-Koehler Publishers, 2021), 6.

32. Taylor, *The Body Is Not an Apology Second Edition: The Power of Radical Self-Love*, 16.

33. Sesali Bowen, "What Women Who Criticize Plastic Surgery Don't See," *New York Times*, March 4, 2020, https://www.nytimes.com/2020/03/04/opinion/black-women-plastic-surgery-natural.html.

34. Germine H. Awad and others, "Beauty and Body Image Concerns Among African American College Women," *The Journal of Black Psychology*, 41, 6 (2015): 540–64, https://doi.org/10.1177/0095798414550864.

35. Jennifer Weiner, "I Feel Personally Judged by J. Lo's Body," *New York Times*, February 4, 2020, https://www.nytimes.com/2020/02/04/opinion/jlo-superbowl-performance.html.

36. Cartner-Morley, "Shades of 50: How the midlife woman went from invisible to the main event."

37. Nicol Natale, "Paulina Porizkova, 55, Says 'Sexy Has No Expiration Date' in Nude Instagram Photo," *Prevention*, February 4, 2021, https://www.prevention.com/life/a35408679/paulina-porizkova-nude-instagram-aging.

38. Elise Solé, "More women over 50 are flaunting their bodies. And that's a good thing, *Yahoo Life*, December 20, 2019, https://www.yahoo.com/now/more-women-over-50-are-flaunting-their-bodies-183709466.html.

39. Dina Spector, "8 Scientifically Proven Reasons Life Is Better If You're Beautiful," *Insider*, June 12, 2013, https://www.businessinsider.com/studies-show-the-advantages-of-being-beautiful-2013-6.

40. Cindy Gallop, phone call to author, January 25, 2021.

41. Taylor, *The Body Is Not an Apology Second Edition: The Power of Radical Self-Love*, 9.

42. Taylor, *The Body Is Not an Apology Second Edition: The Power of Radical Self-Love*, 16.

43. Helen McCrory, "How should a woman live her life?," *The Guardian*, April 16, 2021, https://www.theguardian.com/culture/2021/apr/16/helen-mccrory-how-should-a-woman-live-her-life.

44. Comment on "Older Women Display Their Sexuality—Get Over It," *Fourth Wave*, March 30, 2021, https://medium.com/fourth-wave/older-women-display-their-sexuality-get-over-it-3a5977f36464.

45. Busch, "The Invisibility of Older Women."

46. Anne E. Barrett and Cheryl Robbins, "The multiple sources of women's aging anxiety and their relationship with psychological distress," *Journal of Aging and Health*, 20, 1 (2008): 32–65, https://doi.org/10.1177/0898264307309932.

47. Paige Averett, phone call to author, February 11, 2021.

48. Eden M. Griffin and Karen L. Fingerman, "Online Dating Profile Content of Older Adults Seeking Same- and Cross-Sex Relationships," *Journal of GLBT Family Studies* 14 (2017): 446–66, https://doi.org/10.1080/1550428X.2017.1393362.

49. Silvia Moreno-Domínguez, Tania Raposo, and Paz Elipe, "Body Image and Sexual Dissatisfaction: Differences Among Heterosexual, Bisexual, and Lesbian Women," *Frontiers in Psychology*, 10 (2019): 903, https://doi.org/10.3389/fpsyg.2019.00903.

50. Julie Hale, "Betsey Prioleau: A bewitching new book offers lessons in love," *BookPage*, December 2003, https://bookpage.com/interviews/8231-betsey-prioleau-history#.YEw_-h2IYkg.

51. American Geriatrics Society, "How weight loss is linked to future health for older adults," *ScienceDaily*, September 4, 2018, www.sciencedaily.com/releases/2018/09/180904085124.htm.

52. Meryl Davids Landau, "Oprah's Top Wellness Tips for 2020 and Beyond, *Everyday Health*, January 14, 2020, https://www.everydayhealth.com/healthy-living/oprahs-top-wellness-tips.

53. Pamela Druckerman, *There Are No Grown-Ups: A Midlife Coming-of-Age Story* (New York: Penguin Press, 2018), 86.

54. Lucy Rock, "So now you're middle-aged? Pamela Druckerman can walk you through it," *The Guardian*, May 30, 2018, https://www.theguard

ian.com/society/2018/may/30/pamela-druckerman-there-are-no-grown
-ups-midlife.

55. Keon West, "Naked and Unashamed: Investigations and Applications of the Effects of Naturist Activities on Body Image, Self-Esteem, and Life Satisfaction," *Journal of Happiness Studies* 19 (2018): 677–97, https://doi.org/10.1007/s10902-017-9846-1.

56. Sarah Hardy, "Fashion vs Naturism: Amelia Allen Launches Naked Britain Photography Book via Kehrer Verlag," *FMS*, November 13, 2017, https://fms-mag.com/fashion-vs-naturism-amelia-allen-launches-naked-britain-photography-book-via-kehrer-verlag.

57. V. Pendragon, phone call with author, April 1, 2021.

58. Ela Veresiu, "The #advancedstyle movement celebrates and empowers stylish older women," *The Conversation*, April 19, 2021, https://theconversation.com/the-advancedstyle-movement-celebrates-and-empowers-stylish-older-women-157952.

59. Katie Hunt, "Work, not sex? The real reason Chinese women bound their feet," *CNN*, May 21, 2017, https://www.cnn.com/2017/05/21/health/china-foot-binding-new-theory.

60. Tracy You, "The last foot-binding survivors: Chinese grandmothers uncover their deformed 'lotus feet'—a symbol of beauty less than a century ago," *The Daily Mail*, February 27, 2018, https://www.dailymail.co.uk/news/article-5425801/Last-foot-binding-survivors-captured-beautiful-photos.html.

61. Amanda Foreman, "Why Footbinding Persisted in China for a Millennium," *Smithsonian Magazine*, February 2015, https://www.smithsonianmag.com/history/why-footbinding-persisted-china-millennium-180953971.

62. University of Delaware, "Views of ideal female appearance in China are changing," *Phys.org*, November 28, 2018, https://phys.org/news/2018-11-views-ideal-female-china.html.

63. Rob Schmitz, "China's Marriage Rate Plummets As Women Choose To Stay Single Longer," *NPR*, July 31, 2018, https://www.npr.org/2018/07/31/634048279/chinas-marriage-rate-plummets-as-women-choose-to-stay-single-longer.

64. Maciel and Laganà, "Older women's sexual desire problems: Biopsychosocial factors impacting them and barriers to their clinical assessment."

65. Naomi Wolf, *The Beauty Myth: How Images of Beauty Are Used Against Women* (New York: Harper Perennial, 2002) 186.

66. Taylor, *The Body Is Not an Apology Second Edition: The Power of Radical Self-Love*, 21.

CHAPTER 5

1. Rosalind Wiseman, "Dealing With Grown-Up 'Mean Girls,'" *New York Times*, December 5, 2019, https://www.nytimes.com/2019/12/05/well/family/dealing-with-grown-up-mean-girls.html.

2. Bridget Read, "It's Been 17 Years Since We First Heard About Mean Girls—Have We Learned Anything?," *Vogue*, April 23, 2018, https://www.vogue.com/article/did-we-learn-anything-from-mean-girls-musical-rosa lind-wiseman-queen-bees-wannabees.

3. Emily V. Gordon, "Why Women Compete With Each Other," *New York Times*, October 31, 2015, https://www.nytimes.com/2015/11/01/opinion/sunday/why-women-compete-with-each-other.html.

4. Noam Shpancer, Ph.D., "Feminine Foes: New Science Explores Female Competition," *Psychology Today*, January 26, 2014, https://www.psychologytoday.com/us/blog/insight-therapy/201401/feminine-foes-new-science-explores-female-competition.

5. Lynn Margolies, Ph.D., "Competition Among Women: Myth and Reality," *PsychCentral*, May 17, 2016, https://psychcentral.com/lib/competition-among-women-myth-and-reality#3.

6. Erin Clements, "'Golden Girls' producer Tony Thomas on show's popularity: 'What we built was a family,'" *Today*, June 6, 2019, https://www.today.com/popculture/golden-girls-producer-tony-thomas-show-s-popularity-what-we-t154185.

7. Kath Weston, *Families We Choose: Lesbians, Gays, Kinship (Between Men–between Women)* (New York: Columbia University Press, May 1, 1991).

8. Joe Blevins, "Read This: How The Golden Girls nurtured its considerable gay following," *AV Club*, March 8, 2016, https://www.avclub.com/read-this-how-the-golden-girls-nurtured-its-considerab-1798244966.

9. Amy Blackstone, "Grow Old Like 'The Golden Girls,'" *New York Times*, June 7, 2019, https://www.nytimes.com/2019/06/07/opinion/retirement-aging-golden-girls.html.

10. Bella DePaulo, *How We Live Now: Redefining Home and Family in the 21st Century* (Oregon: Atria Books/Beyond Words, 2015), 183.

11. Julian Beauvais, "Golden Girls: 5 Times Dorothy And Blanche Were Closer Than Sisters (& 5 Times They Were At Each Other's Throats)," *Screen Rant*, April 4, 2021, https://screenrant.com/golden-girls-5-times-dorothy-and-blanche-were-closer-than-sisters-5-times-they-were-at-each-others-throats.

12. Sasha Roseneil, "Foregrounding Friendship: Feminist Pasts, Feminist Futures," In *Handbook of Gender and Women's Studies*, ed. Kathy Davis, Mary Evans, and Judith Lorber (London: SAGE Publications Ltd., 2006) 322–41, http://dx.doi.org/10.4135/9781848608023.n19.

13. McKenzie Jean-Philippe, "How Oprah and Gayle's 45-Year Friendship Began—and Why It's Lasted," *Oprah Daily*, March 4, 2021, https://www.oprahdaily.com/life/relationships-love/a26965035/oprah-and-gayle-friendship.

14. Oprah Winfrey, "Oprah Explains Why She and Gayle King "Will Always be in Each Other's Corner,'" *Oprah Daily*, August 7, 2019, https://www.oprahdaily.com/life/a28323160/oprah-gayle-friendship-memories.

15. Danny Shea, "Oprah Addresses Lesbian Rumors, Cries to Barbara Walters (VIDEO)," *HuffPost,* December 8, 2010, https://www.huffpost.com/entry/oprah-lesbian-rumors-cries-_n_793778.

16. William Deresiewicz, "A Man. A Woman. Just Friends?" *New York Times,* April 8, 2012, https://www.nytimes.com/2012/04/08/opinion/sunday/a-man-a-woman-just-friends.html.

17. Amy Novotney, "The risks of social isolation," *Monitor on Psychology,* 50, 5 (March 2020): 32, https://www.apa.org/monitor/2019/05/ce-corner-isolation.

18. Ashley E. Ermer, Dikla Segel-Karpas, and Jacquelyn J. Benson, "Loneliness trajectories and correlates of social connections among older adult married couples," *JFP: Journal of the Division of Family Psychology of the American Psychological Association* (Division 43), 34, 8, (2020): 1014–24, https://doi.org/10.1037/fam0000652.

19. Elaine O. Cheung, Wendi L. Gardner, and Jason F. Anderson, "Emotionships: Examining People's Emotion-Regulation Relationships and Their Consequences for Well-Being," *Social Psychological and Personality Science* 6, no. 4 (May 2015): 407–14, https://doi.org/10.1177/1948550614564223.

20. Valerie Frankel, "You gotta have friends!," *Self,* October 7, 2009, https://www.self.com/story/how-many-friends-do-you-need.

21. Finkel, Eli J. *The All-Or-Nothing Marriage: How the Best Marriages Work* (New York: Dutton, 2019), 265.

22. Elena Clare Cuffari, "Friendless Women and the Myth of Male Nonage: Why We Need a Better Science of Love and Sex," in *New Philosophies of Sex and Love: Thinking Through Desire,* ed. Sarah LaChance Adams, Christopher M. Davidson, and Caroline R. Lundquist (New York: Rowman & Littlefield Publishers, 2016), 105.

23. Cuffari. "Friendless Women and the Myth of Male Nonage: Why We Need a Better Science of Love and Sex," 106.

24. Shasta Nelson. "Friendships Don't Just Happen!: The Guide to Creating a Meaningful Circle of GirlFriends," *Shastanelson.com,* https://www.shastanelson.com/friendships-dont-just-happen.

25. Laurie A. Rudman and Stephanie A. Goodwin, "Gender differences in automatic in-group bias: Why do women like women more than men like men?," *Journal of Personality and Social Psychology,* 87, 4 (2004): 494–509, https://doi.org/10.1037/0022-3514.87.4.494.

26. Anna Machin and Robin Dunbar, "Sex and Gender as Factors in Romantic Partnerships and Best Friendships," *Journal of Relationships Research* 4 (2013): e8. doi:10.1017/jrr.2013.8.

27. Maria Popova, "Love Undetectable: Andrew Sullivan on Why Friendship Is a Greater Gift Than Romantic Love," *Brain Pickings,* April 23, 2014, https://www.brainpickings.org/2014/04/23/love-undetectable-andrew-sullivan-friendship.

28. Thorne Barrie, "Girls and Boys Together . . . but Mostly Apart: Gender Arrangements in Elementary Schools," in *Relationships and Development,* eds. Willard Hartup and Rubin Zick (New Jersey, Lawrence Erlbaum, 1986): 167–84.

29. Carla D. Brailey and Brittany C. Slatton, "Women, Work, and Inequality in the U.S.: Revisiting the 'Second-Shift,'" *The Journal of Sociology and Social Work* 7 (2019): 1–6.

30. "Gender and Stress," *American Psychological Association,* 2012, https://www.apa.org/news/press/releases/stress/2010/gender-stress.

31. Gale Berkowitz, "UCLA Study on Friendship Among Women," 2002, http://www.anapsid.org/cnd/gender/tendfend.html.

32. Lisa Selin Davis, "Amid an epidemic of loneliness, some friendships grow stronger," *CNN,* October 8, 2020, https://www.cnn.com/2020/10/05/health/fewer-but-stronger-friendships-wellness/index.html.

33. Rosemary Blieszner, Aaron Ogletree, and Rebecca Adams, "Friendship in Later Life: A Research Agenda," *Innovation in Aging,* 3, 1 (2019): igz005, https://doi.org/10.1093/geroni/igz005.

34. Shelley E. Taylor and others, "Behavioral Responses to Stress: Tend and Befriend, Not Fight or Flight," *Psychological Review* 107, 3 (2000): 41–29, https://doi.org/10.1037/0033-295x.107.3.411.

35. Hafford-Letchfield, "Going Solo: Findings from a survey of women ageing without a partner and who do not have children."

36. Anna Muraco and Karen Fredriksen-Goldsen, "'That's what friends do': Informal caregiving for chronically ill midlife and older lesbian, gay, and bisexual adults," *Journal of social and personal relationships,* 28, 8 (2011): 1073–92, https://doi.org/10.1177/0265407511402419.

37. Jacqueline S. Weinstock and Esther D. Rothblum, "Just friends: The role of friendship in lesbians' lives," *Journal of Lesbian Studies,* 22:1 (2018): 1–3, doi:10.1080/10894160.2017.1326762.

38. Jacqueline S. Weinstock, "Lesbian friendships at midlife: Patterns and possibilities for the 21st century," *Journal of Gay & Lesbian Social Services,* 11 (2000): 1–32, doi: 10.1300/j041v11n02_01.

39. Roseneil, "Foregrounding Friendship: Feminist Pasts, Feminist Futures."

40. Rhaina Cohen, "What If Friendship, Not Marriage, Was at the Center of Life?," *The Atlantic,* October 20, 2020, https://www.theatlantic.com/family/archive/2020/10/people-who-prioritize-friendship-over-romance/616779.

41. Elizabeth Brake, "Recognizing Care: The Case for Friendship and Polyamory," *Slace Journal,* 1 (2013), https://slace.syr.edu/issue-1-2013-14-on-equality/recognizing-care-the-case-for-friendship-and-polyamory.

42. Danielle Braff, "From Best Friends to Platonic Spouses," *New York Times,* May 1, 2021, https://www.nytimes.com/2021/05/01/fashion/weddings/from-best-friends-to-platonic-spouses.html.

43. Laura A. Rosenbury, "Friends with Benefits," *Michigan Law Review* 106, (2007): 189, http://scholarship.law.ufl.edu/facultypub/721.

44. Rosenbury, "Friends with Benefits," 233–34.

45. Charlotte Ann Morris, "The significance of friendship in UK single mothers' intimate lives," *Families, Relationships and Societies*, 8, No. 3, (2019), 427–43, https://doi.org/10.1332/204674318X15262010818254.

46. Suzanna M. Rose, "Enjoying the Returns: Women's Friendships After 50," in *Women Over 50*, eds. Varda Muhlbauer and Joan C. Chrisler (Boston: Springer, 2007), 112, https://doi.org/10.1007/978-0-387-46341-4_7.

47. Kayleen Schaefer, *Text Me When You Get Home: The Evolution and Triumph of Modern Female Friendship* (New York: Dutton, 2018), 4.

48. Schaefer, *Text Me When You Get Home: The Evolution and Triumph of Modern Female Friendship*, 6.

49. Andie Nordgren, "The short instructional manifesto for relationship anarchy," *Andie's Log*, July 6, 2012, https://log.andie.se/post/26652940513/the-short-instructional-manifesto-for-relationship.

50. Clare Wiley, "Relationship Anarchy Takes the Judgment Out Of Love," *Medium*, August 6, 2015, https://medium.com/@Clare_Wiley/relationship-anarchy-takes-the-judgment-out-of-love-1c7838e97d3.

51. Bella DePaulo, "If you aren't in a relationship, who is your 'person'?," *Washington Post*, April 4, 2018, https://www.washingtonpost.com/news/soloish/wp/2018/04/04/if-youre-single-who-is-your-person.

52. Anna Muraco and Karen I. Fredriksen-Goldsen, "Turning Points in the Lives of Lesbian and Gay Adults Age 50 and Over," *Advances in Life Course Research*, 30 (2016): 124–32, https://doi.org/10.1016/j.alcr.2016.06.002.

53. Robin Marantz Henig, "The Last Day of Her Life," *New York Times*, May 14, 2015, https://www.nytimes.com/2015/05/17/magazine/the-last-day-of-her-life.html.

54. Matt Richtel, "When an Ex-Spouse Returns as Caregiver," *New York Times*, May 19, 2005, https://www.nytimes.com/2005/05/19/fashion/thursdaystyles/when-an-exspouse-returns-as-caregiver.html.

55. Diane Felmlee and Anna Muraco, "Gender and Friendship Norms Among Older Adults," *Research on Aging*, 31, 3 (2009): 318–44, https://doi.org/10.1177/0164027508330719.

56. Robin Moremen, "Best Friends: The Role of Confidantes in Older Women's Health," *Journal of Women & Aging*, 20 (2008): 149–67, https://doi.org/10.1300/j074v20n01_11.

57. Ashley E. Ermer and Kristin N. Matera, "Older women's friendships: Illuminating the role of marital histories in how older women navigate friendships and caregiving for friends," *Journal of Women & Aging*, 33, 2 (2021): 214–29, https://doi.org/10.1080/08952841.2020.1860632.

58. Rachel Bertsche, *MWF Seeking BFF: My Yearlong Search for a New Best Friend* (New York: Ballantine Books, 2012), 83.

59. Sally Chivers, "How we rely on older adults, especially during the coronavirus pandemic, *The Conversation,* July 30, 2020, https://theconversa tion.com/how-we-rely-on-older-adults-especially-during-the-coronavirus -pandemic-143346.

60. Jeannie Ralston, "Who Are You Calling Invisible?," *Ageist,* January 24, 2019, https://www.weareageist.com/women/who-are-you-calling-invisible.

61. D'Vera Cohn and Jeffrey S. Passel, "A record 64 million Americans live in multigenerational households," *Pew Research Center,* April 5, 2018, https://www.pewresearch.org/fact-tank/2018/04/05/a-record-64-million -americans-live-in-multigenerational-households.

62. Abby Ellin, "New Women's Groups Focus on Generational Mix," *New York Times,* November 10, 2018, https://www.nytimes.com/2018/11/10/ style/intergenerational-womens-groups.html?.

63. "The Positive Impact of Intergenerational Friendships," *AARP Research,* May 2019, https://doi.org/10.26419/res.00314.002.

64. Josephine A Menkin and others, "Positive expectations regarding aging linked to more new friends in later life," *The Journals of Gerontology, Series B: Psychological Sciences and Social Sciences,* 72 (2016): 771–81, https:// doi.org/10.1093/geronb/gbv118.

65. Lise Funderburg, "The Two Friends Every Woman Needs," *Good Housekeeping,* January 25, 2012, https://www.goodhousekeeping.com/life/ inspirational-stories/a19612/long-lasting-friendships.

66. Marcella Runell Hall and Kersha Smith, editors, *UnCommon Bonds: Women Reflect on Race and Friendship* (Switzerland: Peter Lang Inc., International Academic Publishers, 2018), 3.

67. Karen S. Rook, "Gaps in Social Support Resources in Later Life: An Adaptational Challenge in Need of Further Research," *Journal of social and personal relationships,* 26, 1 (2009): 103–12, https://doi .org/10.1177/0265407509105525.

68. Hall and Smith, *UnCommon Bonds: Women Reflect on Race and Friendship,* 14.

69. Lindsay Dunsmuir, "Many Americans have no friends of another race: poll," *Reuters,* August 7, 2013, https://www.reuters.com/article/us -usa-poll-race/many-americans-have-no-friends-of-another-race-poll-idUS BRE97704320130808.

70. Deborah L. Plummer and others, "Patterns of Adult Cross-Racial Friendships: A Context for Understanding Contemporary Race Relations," *Cultural Diversity and Ethnic Minority Psychology,* 22, 4 (2016): 479–94, https:// doi.org/10.1037/cdp0000079.

71. Dudley L. Poston Jr. and Rogelio Sáenz, "The US white majority will soon disappear forever," *The Conversation,* April 30, 2019, https://theconver sation.com/the-us-white-majority-will-soon-disappear-forever-115894.

72. G. Clare Wenger and Vanessa Burholt, "Changes in levels of social isolation and loneliness among older people in a rural area: A twenty-year

longitudinal study," *Canadian Journal on Aging, La Revue Canadienne du Vieillissement*, 23, 2 (2004): 115–27, https://doi.org/10.1353/cja.2004.0028.

73. Ian Sample, "Smiling Scots, worried Welsh and lazy Londoners: Survey maps regional personality types," *The Guardian*, March 24, 2015, https://www.theguardian.com/science/2015/mar/25/survey-maps-regional-personality-types.

74. DePaulo, "If you aren't in a relationship, who is your 'person?'"

75. Frankel, "You gotta have friends!"

76. Diane Felmlee and Anna Muraco, "Gender and Friendship Norms Among Older Adults," *Research on Aging*, 31, 3 (2009): 318–44, https://doi.org/10.1177/0164027508330719.

77. Rebecca G. Adams and Rosemary Blieszner, "Structural Predictors of Problematic Friendships in Later Life," *Personal Relationships*, 5 (1998): 439–447, https://doi.org/10.1111/j.1475-6811.1998.tb00181.x.

78. Blieszner, Ogletree, and Adams, "Friendship in Later Life: A Research Agenda."

79. Robin D. Moremen, "The Downside of Friendship: Sources of Strain in Older Women's Friendships," *Journal of Women & Aging*, 20: 1–2, (2008): 169–87, https://doi.org/10.1300/j074v20n01_12.

CHAPTER 6

1. Ursula K. Le Guin, *Dancing at the Edge of the World: Thoughts on Words, Women, Places* (New York: Grove Press, 2017), 5.

2. Janice Kaplan, *The Genius of Women From Overlooked to Changing the World* (New York: Dutton, 2021), 167.

3. Michael T. Vale, Toni L. Bisconti, and Jennifer F. Sublett, "Benevolent ageism: Attitudes of overaccommodative behavior toward older women," *The Journal of Social Psychology*, 160, 5, (2020): 548–58, DOI: 10.1080/00224545.2019.1695567.

4. Muriel Dumont, Marie Sarlet, and Benoit Dardenne, "Be Too Kind to a Woman, She'll Feel Incompetent: Benevolent Sexism Shifts Self-construal and Autobiographical Memories Toward Incompetence," *Sex Roles*. 62 (2020): 545–53. 10.1007/s11199-008-9582-4.

5. Linda P. Fried, and others, "Frailty in older adults: Evidence for a phenotype," *The Journals of Gerontology Series A*, 56, 3 (2001): M146–M156, https://doi.org/10.1093/gerona/56.3.m146.

6. Joan Chrisler, Angela Barney, and Brigida Palatino, "Ageism Can be Hazardous to Women's Health: Ageism, Sexism, and Stereotypes of Older Women in the Healthcare System," *Journal of Social Issues* 72 (2016): 86–104. 10.1111/josi.12157.

7. Laura Kiesel, "Women and pain: Disparities in experience and treatment," *Harvard Health,* October 09, 2017, https://www.health.harvard .edu/blog/women-and-pain-disparities-in-experience-and-treatment -2017100912562.

8. Ashton Applewhite, *This Chair Rocks: A Manifesto Against Ageism* (New York: Celadon Books, 2019), 89.

9. J. Dianne Garner, "Feminism and feminist gerontology," *Journal of Women & Aging,* 11 (1999): 3–12, https://doi.org/10.1300/J074v11n02_02.

10. Chrisler, Barney, and Palatino, "Ageism Can be Hazardous to Women's Health: Ageism, Sexism, and Stereotypes of Older Women in the Healthcare System."

11. David Robson, "The age you feel means more than your actual birthdate," *BBC Future,* July 19, 2018, https://www.bbc.com/future/ article/20180712-the-age-you-feel-means-more-than-your-actual-birthdate.

12. Oregon State University. "'Aging well' greatly affected by hopes and fears for later life," *ScienceDaily,* January 21, 2021, www.sciencedaily.com/ releases/2021/01/210121150929.htm.

13. Joan Chrisler, "Teaching Taboo Topics: Menstruation, Menopause, and the Psychology of Women, *Psychology of Women Quarterly,* 37 (2013): 128–32, 10.1177/0361684312471326.

14. Arline T. Geronimus and others, "Do US Black Women Experience Stress-Related Accelerated Biological Aging?: A Novel Theory and First Population-Based Test of Black-White Differences in Telomere Length," *Human Nature* 21, 1 (2010): 19–38, https://doi.org/10.1007/s12110-010-9078-0.

15. Zinzi D. Bailey and others, "Structural racism and health inequities in the USA: Evidence and interventions," *Lancet,* 389, 10077 (2017): 1453–63, doi: 10.1016/S0140-6736 (17) 30569-X. PMID: 28402827.

16. Danielle L. Beatty, and others, "Everyday Discrimination Prospectively Predicts Inflammation Across 7 Years in Racially Diverse Midlife Women: Study of Women's Health Across the Nation," *The Journal of Social Issues,* 70, 2 (2014): 298–314, https://doi.org/10.1111/josi.12061.

17. Eleanor Mills, "I was told at Facebook I was middle-aged at 35," *The Daily Mail,* June 16, 2021, https://www.dailymail.co.uk/femail/ article-9693729/Sheryl-Sandberg-talks-finding-love-fighting-women-hit -pandemic.html.

18. Dr. Jen Gunter, "Women Can Have a Better Menopause. Here's How," *New York Times,* May 25, 2021, https://www.nytimes.com/2021/05/25/ opinion/feminist-menopause.html.

19. Lisa Selin Davis, "Why Modern Medicine Keeps Overlooking Menopause," *New York Times,* April 6, 2021, https://www.nytimes .com/2021/04/06/us/menopause-perimenopause-symptoms.html.

20. Adriana Velez, "Menopause Is Different for Women of Color," *EndocrineWeb,* March 10, 2021, https://www.endocrineweb.com/menopause -different-women-color.

21. "Childless women more likely to begin menopause early, study finds," *National Child Development Study*, January 25, 2017, https://ncds.info/childless-women-more-likely-to-begin-menopause-early-study-finds.

22. Carol B. Vandenakker and Dorothea D. Glass, "Menopause and aging with disability," *Physical medicine and rehabilitation clinics of North America*, 12, 1 (2001): 133–51, https://doi.org/10.1016/S1047-9651(18)30087-1.

23. Chrisler, "Teaching Taboo Topics: Menstruation, Menopause, and the Psychology of Women."

24. Beverley Ayers, Mark Forshaw, and Myra S. Hunter, "The impact of attitudes towards the menopause on women's symptom experience: A systematic review," *Maturitas*, 65, 1 (2010): 28–36, https://doi.org/10.1016/j.maturitas.2009.10.016.

25. Sharon J. Parish and others, "The MATE survey: Men's perceptions and attitudes towards menopause and their role in partners' menopausal transition," *Menopause*, 26, 10 (2019): 1110–16, doi: 10.1097/GME.0000000000001373.

26. Parish, "The MATE survey: Men's perceptions and attitudes towards menopause and their role in partners' menopausal transition."

27. Janice P. Nimura, "Why 'Unwell Women' Have Gone Misdiagnosed for Centuries," review of *Unwell Women: Misdiagnosis and Myth in a Man-Made World* by Elinor Cleghorn, *New York Times*, June 8, 2021, https://www.nytimes.com/2021/06/08/books/review/unwell-women-elinor-cleghorn.html.

28. Mary Elizabeth Williams, "'Unwell Women' author Elinor Cleghorn: Women's pain 'isn't taken seriously' by doctors," *Salon*, June 8, 2021, https://www.salon.com/2021/06/08/unwell-women-author-elinor-cleghorn-womens-pain-isnt-taken-seriously-by-doctors.

29. Elinor Cleghorn, *Unwell Women: Misdiagnosis and Myth in a Man-Made World* (New York: Dutton, 2021), 307, 313.

30. Cleghorn, *Unwell Women: Misdiagnosis and Myth in a Man-Made World*, 306.

31. Cleghorn, *Unwell Women: Misdiagnosis and Myth in a Man-Made World*, 13.

32. Williams, "'Unwell Women' author Elinor Cleghorn: Women's pain 'isn't taken seriously' by doctors."

33. Chrisler, "Ageism can be Hazardous to Women's Health: Ageism, Sexism, and Stereotypes of Older Women in the Healthcare System."

34. University of Miami, "Women's pain not taken as seriously as men's pain: A new study suggests that when men and women express the same amount of pain, women's pain is considered less intense based on gender stereotypes," *ScienceDaily*, www.sciencedaily.com/releases/2021/04/210406164124.htm.

35. Centers for Disease Control and Prevention, "Atlas Plus: HIV, Hepatitis, STD, TB, Social Determinants of Health Data," 2018, https://gis.cdc.gov/grasp/nchhstpatlas/charts.html.

36. Centers for Disease Control and Prevention, "Sexually Transmitted Disease Surveillance 2019: Reported STDs in the U.S. reach all-time high for 6th consecutive year," April 13, 2021, https://www.cdc.gov/std/statistics/2019/default.htm.

37. Elaine K. Howley, "What to Know About Rising STD Rates Among Seniors," *U.S. News*, December 10, 2018, https://health.usnews.com/health-care/patient-advice/articles/2018-12-10/what-to-know-about-rising-std-rates-among-seniors.

38. Matthew Lee Smith and others, "Sexually Transmitted Infection Knowledge among Older Adults: Psychometrics and Test-Retest Reliability," *International Journal of Environmental Research and Public Health*, 17, 7 (2020): 2462, https://doi.org/10.3390/ijerph17072462.

39. Carrie A. Karvonen-Gutierrez, "The importance of disability as a health issue for mid-life women," *Women's Midlife Health* 1, 10 (2015), https://doi.org/10.1186/s40695-015-0011-x.

40. Toni Calasanti and Neal King, "Successful Aging, Ageism, and the Maintenance of Age and Gender Relations," in *Successful Aging as a Contemporary Obsession: Global Perspectives*, ed. Sarah Lamb (New Jersey: Rutgers University Press, 2017) 27–40.

41. Leigh Ann Hubbard, "Martha Holstein: Feminism and the Future of Aging," *Silver Century Foundation*, March 8, 2018, https://www.silvercentury.org/2018/03/martha-holstein-feminism-and-the-future-of-aging.

42. Sara M. Hofmeier and others, "Body image, aging, and identity in women over 50: The Gender and Body Image (GABI) study," *Journal of Women & Aging*, 29, 1 (2017): 3–14, https://doi.org/10.1080/08952841.2015.1065140.

43. Natalie J. Sabik, "Ageism and Body Esteem: Associations With Psychological Well-Being Among Late Middle-Aged African American and European American Women," *The Journals of Gerontology: Series B*, 70, 2 (2015): 189–199, https://doi.org/10.1093/geronb/gbt080.

44. Abigail T. Brooks, "Opting In or Opting Out?: North American Women Share Strategies for Aging Successfully with (and Without) Cosmetic Intervention," in *Successful Aging as a Contemporary Obsession: Global Perspectives*, ed. Sarah Lamb (New Jersey: Rutgers University Press, 2017), 41–54.

45. Margaret Morganroth Gullette, *Declining to Decline: Cultural Combat and the Politics of the Midlife* (Virginia: University Press of Virginia Charlottesville, 1997).

46. Tamara A. Baker and others, "Reconceptualizing Successful Aging Among Black Women and the Relevance of the Strong Black Woman Archetype," *The Gerontologist*, 55, 1 (2015): 51–57, https://doi.org/10.1093/geront/gnu105.

47. Jennifer M Jabson Tree and others, "What Is Successful Aging in Lesbian and Bisexual Women? Application of the Aging-Well Model," *The Journals of Gerontology: Series B* (2020): gbaa130, https://doi.org/10.1093/geronb/gbaa130.

48. Harry Herrick, Karen J. Luken, and Pam Dickens, "Women with disabilities and heart disease (North Carolina BRFSS Surveillance Update No. 5)," Raleigh, NC: State Center for Health Statistics, North Carolina Division of Public Health, 2011, https://fpg.unc.edu/sites/fpg.unc.edu/files/resources/reports-and-policy-briefs/SurveillanceUpdate5_WomenWithDisabilitiesAndHeartDisease_2011.pdf.

49. Margaret Nosek and others, "Study of Women With Physical Disabilities: Final Report," *Sexuality and Disability* 19 (2001): 5–40, 10.1023/A:1010716820677.

50. Margaret Nosek, "The Changing Face of Women with Disabilities: Are We Ready?" *Journal of Women's Health*, 15, 9 (2006): 996–99, https://doi.org/10.1089/jwh.2006.15.996.

51. Sara Radin, "Queer Crip Fashion: For Standing Out, Proudly," *Refinery*, 29, July 24, 2021, https://www.refinery29.com/en-us/2020/07/9921895/queer-crip-fashion-disability-rebirth.

52. Shivani Chinnappan, "Long COVID: The Impact on Women and Ongoing Research," *Society for Women's Health Research*, March 18, 2021, https://swhr.org/long-covid-the-impact-on-women-and-ongoing-research.

53. Jennifer M. Ortman, Victoria A. Velkoff, and Howard Hogan, "An Aging Nation: The Older Population in the United States," U.S. Census Bureau, May 2014, https://www.census.gov/prod/2014pubs/p25-1140.pdf.

54. Jennifer Burgmann, "Why I'm Afraid of Aging With a Disability," *The Mighty*, February 17, 2020, https://www.yahoo.com/now/why-im-afraid-aging-disability-224042506.html.

CHAPTER 7

1. https://www.gq.com/story/beyonce-cover-story-interview-gq-february-2013.

2. Neha Thirani Bagrim, "New research confirms the 'sexuality pay gap' is real," *Quartz*, January 12, 2017, https://qz.com/881303/eight-million-americans-are-affected-by-a-pay-gap-that-no-one-talks-about.

3. Robin Bleiweis, "Quick Facts About the Gender Wage Gap," *Center for American Progress*, March 24, 2020, https://www.americanprogress.org/issues/women/reports/2020/03/24/482141/quick-facts-gender-wage-gap.

4. Asaf Levanon, Paula England, and Paul Allison, "Occupational Feminization and Pay: Assessing Causal Dynamics Using 1950–2000 U.S. Census Data," *Social Forces*, 88, 2 (2009): 865–91, https://doi.org/10.1353/sof.0.0264.

5. Jill Yavorsky and Janette Dill, "Unemployment and men's entrance into female-dominated jobs," *Social Science Research*, 85 (2020): 102–373, doi:10.1016/j.ssresearch.2019.102373.

6. Terry Arendell, "Reflections on the Researcher–Researched Relationship: A Woman Interviewing Men," *Qualitative Sociology*, 20, 3 (1997): 341–68, https://doi.org/10.1023/A:1024727316052.

7. Katie McLaughlin, "5 things women couldn't do in the 1960s," *CNN*, August 25, 2014, https://www.cnn.com/2014/08/07/living/sixties-women-5-things.

8. Michael Gold, "Helping Women Overcome Society's Outdated Messages on Money," *New York Times*, June 17, 2019, https://www.nytimes.com/2019/06/17/business/sallie-krawcheck-stephanie-cohen-new-rules.html.

9. Maurie Backman, "A Summary of 20 Years of Research and Statistics on Women in Investing," *The Motley Fool*, March 4, 2021, https://www.fool.com/research/women-in-investing-research.

10. Barbara Stanny, "Money Coach and Author." Interview by Farnoosh Torabi, *So Money*, February 13, 2015, Audio, 31.25, https://podcast.farnoosh.tv/episode/barbara-stanny/.

11. Farnoosh Torabi, "Wives: Stop Leaving Money Management to Your Spouse," *Bloomberg*, November 14, 2020, https://www.bloomberg.com/opinion/articles/2020-11-14/personal-finance-advice-for-women-avoiding-money-in-marriage.

12. Kate Levinson, *Emotional Currency: A Woman's Guide to Building a Healthy Relationship With Money* (California: Celestial Arts, 2011) 1, 94.

13. Renee Stepler, "Led by Baby Boomers, divorce rates climb for America's 50+ population," Pew Research Center, March 9, 2017, https://www.pewresearch.org/fact-tank/2017/03/09/led-by-baby-boomers-divorce-rates-climb-for-americas-50-population.

14. UBS, "Own Your Worth 2021: Building bridges, breaking barriers," May 6, 2021, http://www.static-ubs.com/content/dam/assets/wma/us/documents/own-your-worth-building-bridges-Q221-us-en.pdf.

15. Kerry Fristoe, "Robin Hauser Wants Women to Get Savvy About Their Personal Finances," *Lioness Magazine*, March 31, 2021, https://lionessmagazine.com/robin-hauser-wants-women-to-get-savvy-about-their-personal-financess.

16. Robin Hauser, phone call to author, May 14, 2020.

17. Eugenie Allen, "Get Back to Work," review of *The Feminine Mistake*, by Leslie Bennetts, *New York Times*, May 6, 2007, https://www.nytimes.com/2007/05/06/books/review/Allen.t.html.

18. Rebecca Mead, "The Wives of Others," review of *The Feminine Mistake*, by Leslie Bennetts, *New York Times*, April 16, 2007, https://www.newyorker.com/magazine/2007/04/16/the-wives-of-others)

19. Barbara A. Butrica and Karen E. Smith, "The Retirement Prospects of Divorced Women," *Social Security Bulletin*, 72, 1 (2012): 11–22, https://www.ssa.gov/policy/docs/ssb/v72n1/v72n1p11.html.

20. Kathleen Michon, "How Much Will My Divorce Cost and How Long Will It Take?," *Nolo*, 2019, https://www.nolo.com/legal-encyclopedia/ctp/cost-of-divorce.html.

21. Kristin Smith, "Recessions Accelerate Trend of Wives as Breadwinners," *Carsey Institute*, 56 (2012), https://scholars.unh.edu/cgi/viewcontent.cgi?referer=https://www.google.com/&httpsredir=1&article=1180&context=carsey; Andrew L. Yarrow, "I spoke to hundreds of American men who still can't find work," *Vox*, September 17, 2018, https://www.vox.com/first-person/2018/9/15/17859134/recession-financial-crisis-2018-men.

22. Kim Parker, Rachel Minkin, and Jesse Bennett, "Economic Fallout From COVID-19 Continues to Hit Lower-Income Americans the Hardest," Pew Research Center, September 24, 2020, https://www.pewresearch.org/social-trends/2020/09/24/economic-fallout-from-covid-19-continues-to-hit-lower-income-americans-the-hardest.

23. C. Nicole Mason and Alicia Modestino, "'Shecession': The Pandemic's Impact On Women in the Workforce," interview by Meghna Chakrabarti, *On Point*, WBUR, October 22, 2020, audio, 47:18, https://www.wbur.org/onpoint/2020/10/22/shecession-the-pandemics-impact-on-women-in-the-workplace.

24. Soraya Chemaly, "Coronavirus could hurt women the most. Here's how to prevent a patriarchal pandemic," *Think*, April 20, 2020, https://www.nbcnews.com/think/opinion/coronavirus-could-hurt-women-most-here-s-how-prevent-patriarchal-ncna1186581.

25. Erin Schumaker, "What we know about coronavirus' long-term effects," *ABC News*, April 17, 2020, https://abcnews.go.com/Health/coronavirus-long-term-effects/story?id=69811566.

26. D'Vera Cohn, Gretchen Livingston, and Wendy Wang, "After Decades of Decline, A Rise in Stay-at-Home Mothers," *Pew Research Center*, April 8, 2014, https://www.pewresearch.org/social-trends/2014/04/08/after-decades-of-decline-a-rise-in-stay-at-home-mothers.

27. Karen Karbo, "The Accidental Breadwinner," *New York Times*, December 12, 2008, https://www.nytimes.com/2008/12/14/fashion/14love.html.

28. UBS, "New UBS report reveals that joint financial participation is the key to gender equality," July 6, 2020, https://www.ubs.com/global/en/media/display-page-ndp/en-20200706-key-to-gender-equality.html.

29. Karbo, "The Accidental Breadwinner."

30. Erica Tempesta, "Paulina Porizkova says she regrets allowing late husband Ric Ocasek to manage her money, saying it gave him total 'control' over her life—and made others view her as nothing more than 'the vapid wife of a rockstar,'" *The Daily Mail*, March 2, 2021, https://www.dailymail.co.uk/femail/article-9317873/Paulina-Porizkova-regrets-giving-late-husband-Ric-Ocasek-control-money.html.

31. Tempesta, "Paulina Porizkova."

32. Kim Parker and Renee Stepler, "Americans see men as the financial providers, even as women's contributions grow," *Pew Research Center*, September 20, 2017, https://www.pewresearch.org/fact-tank/2017/09/20/americans-see-men-as-the-financial-providers-even-as-womens-contributions-grow.

33. Lydia Saad, "Children a Key Factor in Women's Desire to Work Outside the Home," *Gallup*, October 7, 2015, https://news.gallup.com/poll/186050/children-key-factor-women-desire-work-outside-home.aspx.

34. Darlena Cunha, "I'm One of the 56% of American Mothers Who 'Prefer' to Stay Home," *Time*, October 9, 2015, https://time.com/4068559/gallup-poll-stay-at-home-mothers.

35. Cohn, Livingston, and Wang, "After Decades of Decline, A Rise in Stay-at-Home Mothers."

36. Jo Boaler, "Parents' Beliefs about Math Change Their Children's Achievement," *YouCubed*, https://www.youcubed.org/resources/parents-beliefs-math-change-childrens-achievement.

37. Hiroshima University, "Some women's retirement plan: Rely on Prince Charming," *ScienceDaily*, www.sciencedaily.com/releases/2016/06/160622102127.htm.

38. Nicole Maestas, "The Return to Work and Women's Employment Decisions," *National Bureau of Economic Research Working Paper no. 24429* (March 2018), DOI 10.3386/w24429.

39. Alina Tugend "When Only One Spouse Retires," *Kiplinger*, November 20, 2020, https://www.kiplinger.com/retirement/601791/when-only-one-spouse-retires.

40. Jennifer Barrett, "Here's One More Way Women Get Shortchanged on Money Matters," *The Daily Beast*, May. 16, 2021, https://www.thedailybeast.com/heres-one-more-way-women-get-shortchanged-on-money-matters.

41. Kara I. Stevens, "4 Ways 'Strong Black Woman Syndrome' Keeps Us Poor," *Ebony*, December 11, 2019, https://www.ebony.com/career-finance/4-ways-strongblack-woman-syndrome-keeps-us-poor-444.

42. Sarah Jane Glynn, "Breadwinning Mothers Continue to Be the U.S. Norm," *Center for American Progress*, May 10, 2019, https://www.americanprogress.org/issues/women/reports/2019/05/10/469739/breadwinning-mothers-continue-u-s-norm.

43. Jennifer L. Barrett, *Think Like a Breadwinner: A Wealth-Building Manifesto for Women Who Want to Earn More (and Worry Less)* (New York: G.P. Putnam's Sons, 2021), 12.

44. "The Prince Charming syndrome," *New Zealand Herald*, April 16, 2004, https://www.nzherald.co.nz/nz/the-prince-charming-syndrome/HCYHB2HHZBJJ4DVXXZM2L5GTRA.

45. "Wage Gap May Help Explain Why More Women Are Anxious and Depressed Than Men," *Columbia Mailman School of Health*, January 5, 2016,

https://www.publichealth.columbia.edu/public-health-now/news/wage
-gap-may-help-explain-why-more-women-are-anxious-and-depressed-men.

46. "Women & Financial Wellness: Beyond the Bottom Line," *Merrill Lynch and Age Wave*, (2019), https://www.bofaml.com/content/dam/boam limages/documents/articles/ID18_0244/ml_womens_study.pdf.

47. Benjamin Artz, Amanda Goodall, and Andrew J. Oswald, "Research: Women Ask for Raises as Often as Men, but Are Less Likely to Get Them," *Harvard Business Review*, June 25, 2018, https://hbr.org/2018/06/research -women-ask-for-raises-as-often-as-men-but-are-less-likely-to-get-them.

48. Butrica and Smith, "The Retirement Prospects of Divorced Women."

49. Jonathan Van Meter, "How Kris Jenner Is Taking the Kardashian-Jenner Empire to Hulu and Beyond," *Wall Street Journal Magazine*, March 23, 2021, https://www.wsj.com/articles/kris-jenner-interview-kardashian-kim -kanye-chrissy-11616502549.

50. Christine Platt, "Learning to Love and Let Go: What My Divorce Taught Me About Living With Less," *Real Simple*, June 4, 2021, https:// www.realsimple.com/home-organizing/organizing/what-divorce-taught -me-about-decluttering.

51. Christine Platt, *The Afrominimalist's Guide to Living with Less* (New York: Tiller Press, 2021), 7.

52. Teronda Seymore, "Practical Ways a Minimalist Lifestyle Frees Your Mind & Your Money," *XO Necole*, January 3, 2020, https://www.xonecole .com/minimalist-lifestyle-saves-money.

53. Sara Goudarzi, "Men as Addicted to Shopping as Women," *Live Science*, September 30, 2006, https://www.livescience.com/1036-men-addicted -shopping-women.html.

54. Kathy Gottberg, "Rightsizing Your Finances—A SMART Way to Manage Money," *SMART Living 365*, https://www.smartliving365.com/ rightsizing-your-finances-a-smart-way-to-manage-money.

55. Danielle C. Cath and others, "Age-Specific Prevalence of Hoarding and Obsessive-Compulsive Disorder: A Population-Based Study," *The American Journal of Geriatric Psychiatry*, 25, 3 (2017): 245–55, https://doi .org/10.1016/j.jagp.2016.11.006.

56. Levinson, *Emotional Currency: A Woman's Guide to Building a Healthy Relationship With Money*, 16.

57. Stanny, interview.

58. Angie O'Leary, "Opinion: When women control the wealth, society reaps the benefits, *MarketWatch*, January 4, 2019, https://www.market watch.com/story/when-women-control-the-wealth-society-reaps-the-bene fits-2019-01-04.

59. Gary Mottola, "Gender, Generation and Financial Knowledge: A Six-Year Perspective," *FINRA Investor Education Foundation*, March 2018, https:// www.usfinancialcapability.org/downloads/Issue-Brief-Gender-Generation -and-Financial-Knowledge-A-Six-Year-Perspective.pdf.

60. Fritz Gilbert, "What Baby Boomer Women Need to Know About Their Finances," *The Retirement Manifesto,* July 4, 2017, https://www.the retirementmanifesto.com/what-baby-boomer-women-need-to-know-about -their-finances.

61. Tamara Gillan, "Why are the majority of women struggling with self-esteem issues?," *StartUps Magazine,* https://startupsmagazine.co.uk/article -why-are-majority-women-struggling-self-esteem-issues.

62. Kerry Hannon, "Opinion: This is why so many women face poverty in their old age," *MarketWatch,* September 29, 2020, https://www.market watch.com/story/this-is-why-so-many-women-face-poverty-in-their-old -age-2020-09-29.

63. Michelle Fox, "How women can take control of their money and grow their wealth, *CNBC,* September 6, 2019, https://www.cnbc.com/2019/09/06/ how-women-can-take-control-of-their-money-and-grow-their-wealth.html.

64. Farnoosh Torabi, "I've been writing about money for 15 years, and here are the 9 best pieces of financial advice I can give you," *Insider,* October 7, 2015, https://www.businessinsider.com/personal-finance/best-money -advice-farnoosh-torabi-2015-10#-2.

65. Judy Strauss, "The Baby Boomers Meet Menopause: Fertility, Attractiveness, and Affective Response to the Menopausal Transition," *Sex Roles* 68 (2013): 77–90, https://doi.org/10.1007/s11199-011-0002-9.

CHAPTER 8

1. Norma Kamali, *Norma Kamali: I Am Invincible* (New York: Harry N. Abrams, 2011).

2. Kaplan, *The Genius of Women From Overlooked to Changing the World,* 6.

3. Rebecca Knight, "Balancing feminism with caring about what I look like," *Motherwell,* May 13, 2020, https://motherwellmag.com/2020/05/13/ balancing-feminism-with-caring-about-what-i-look-like/.

4. Leah Dolan, "Teens are worried about wrinkles. Here's how Gen Z is helping to fuel a beauty boom," CNN, May 6, 2021, https://www.cnn.com/ style/article/anti-aging-trend-teens/index.html.

5. Dolan, "Teens are worried about wrinkles. Here's how Gen Z is helping to fuel a beauty boom."

6. Anna Rosa Donizzetti, "Ageism in an Aging Society: The Role of Knowledge, Anxiety about Aging, and Stereotypes in Young People and Adults," *International journal of environmental research and public health,* 16, 8 (2019): 1329, https://doi.org/10.3390/ijerph16081329.

7. Donizzetti, "Ageism in an Aging Society: The Role of Knowledge, Anxiety about Aging, and Stereotypes in Young People and Adults."

8. Stefania Medetti, "Battle the stigma of old age and keep passion alive," *The Age Buster*, August 28, 2019, https://www.theagebuster.com/blog-page/2019/8/28/battle-the-stigma-of-old-age-and-keep-passion-alive.

9. Gaby Hinsliff, "'A weird liberation': Why women are exposing the wild truth about midlife and menopause," *The Guardian*, September 22, 2020, https://www.theguardian.com/lifeandstyle/2020/sep/22/weird-liberation-women-wild-truth-midlife-menopause.

10. Richard A. Settersten Jr., "Some Things I Have Learned About Aging by Studying the Life Course," *Innovation in Aging*, 1, 2 (2017): igx014, https://doi.org/10.1093/geroni/igx014.

11. Rainesford Stauffer, "Ageism Hurts All of Us, Even 'Young People,'" *Elle*, May 6, 2021, https://www.elle.com/life-love/a36290047/ageism-hurts-all-of-us-even-young-people.

Bibliography

Adams, Rebecca G., and Rosemary Blieszner. "Structural Predictors of Problematic Friendships in Later Life," *Personal Relationships*, 5 (1998): 439–37. https://doi.org/10.1111/j.1475-6811.1998.tb00181.x.

"Ageism: The Last Acceptable Prejudice in America | Real Time with Bill Maher (HBO)," November 7, 2014. Video 5:57. https://www.youtube.com/watch?v=0kWaKhrpa28.

"Aging baby boomers, childless and unmarried, at risk of becoming 'elder orphans,'" *Eureka Alert*, May 15, 2015. https://www.eurekalert.org/pub_releases/2015-05/nsij-abb051315.php.

Aging Without Children Consultancy, March 15, 2021. https://ageingwithoutchildrenconsultancy.com/2021/02/25/the-invisibility-of-people-with-out-children-is-a-life-course-issue-which-has-a-drastic-impact-on-policy-around-age-and-ageing.

Allen, Amelia, *Naked Britain*. Germany: Kehrer Verlag, 2017.

American Geriatrics Society. "How weight loss is linked to future health for older adults," *ScienceDaily*, September 4, 2018. www.sciencedaily.com/releases/2018/09/180904085124.htm.

American Society of Plastic Surgeons. "2018 Plastic Surgery Statistics Report." https://www.plasticsurgery.org/documents/News/Statistics/2018/plastic-surgery-statistics-full-report-2018.pdf.

American Sociological Association. "Women more likely than men to initiate divorces, but not non-marital breakups," *ScienceDaily*, www.sciencedaily.com/releases/2015/08/150822154900.htm.

Amoratis, Pandora. "Go au naturale! From letting nails breathe to air drying hair like Ariana Grande, beauty experts reveal why it's a good idea to embrace the natural look while in quarantine." *The Daily Mail*, April 16, 2020. https://www.dailymail.co.uk/femail/article-8221941/Beauty-experts-reveal-look-better-later.html.

Anderson, Lisa. "It's official: Many women become invisible after 49." *Thomson Reuters Foundation.* April 13, 2015. https://www.reuters.com/ar ticle/us-rights-women-ageing/its-official-many-women-become-invisible -after-49-idUSKBN0N41RH20150413.

Andrews, Molly. "Ageful and proud," *Ageing and Society,* 20, no. 6 (November 2000): 791–95.

Appelo, Tim. "Geena Davis Calls Hollywood's Age Bias 'Dismal.'" *AARP,* November 4, 2020. https://www.aarp.org/entertainment/movies-for -grownups/info-2020/geena-davis-actresses-ageism-in-hollywood.html.

Applewhite, Ashton, *This Chair Rocks: A Manifesto Against Ageism.* New York: Celadon Books, 2019.

Arendell, Terry. "Reflections on the Researcher–Researched Relationship: A Woman Interviewing Men." *Qualitative Sociology,* 20, 3 (1997): 341–68. https://doi.org/10.1023/A:1024727316052.

Artz, Benjamin, Amanda Goodall, and Andrew J. Oswald. "Research: Women Ask for Raises as Often as Men, but Are Less Likely to Get Them." *Harvard Business Review,* June 25. 2018. https://hbr.org/2018/06/research -women-ask-for-raises-as-often-as-men-but-are-less-likely-to-get-them.

Atkins, David C., Donald H. Baucom, and Neil S. Jacobson. "Understanding infidelity: Correlates in a national random sample." *Journal of Family Psychology,* 15(4) (2001): 735–49. https://doi.org/10.1037/0893-3200.15.4.735.

Averett, Paige, Intae Yoon, and Carol L. Jenkins. "Older lesbian sexuality: Identity, sexual behavior, and the impact of aging." *Journal of sex research,* 49(5) (2012): 495–507. https://doi.org/10.1080/00224499.2011.582543.

Awad, Germine H., C. Norwood, D. S. Taylor, M. Martinez, S. McClain, B. Jones, A. Holman, and C. Chapman-Hilliard. "Beauty and Body Image Concerns Among African American College Women." *The Journal of Black Psychology,* 41, 6 (2015): 540–64. https://doi.org/10.1177/0095798414550864.

Ayers, Beverley, Mark Forshaw, and Myra S. Hunter. "The impact of attitudes towards the menopause on women's symptom experience: A systematic review." *Maturitas,* 65, 1 (2010): 28–36. https://doi.org/10.1016/j .maturitas.2009.10.016.

Backman, Maurie. "A Summary of 20 Years of Research and Statistics on Women in Investing." *The Motley Fool,* March 4, 2021. https://www.fool .com/research/women-in-investing-research.

Bagrim, Neha Thirani. "New research confirms the 'sexuality pay gap' is real." *Quartz,* January 12, 2017. https://qz.com/881303/eight-million -americans-are-affected-by-a-pay-gap-that-no-one-talks-about.

Bailey, Moya, *Misogynoir Transformed: Black Women's Digital Resistance.* New York: New York University Press, 2021.

Bailey, Zinzi D., Nancy Krieger, Madina Agénor, Jasmine Graves, Natalia Linos, Mary T. Bassett. "Structural racism and health inequities in the USA: Evidence and interventions." *Lancet,* 389, 10077 (2017): 1453–63. doi: 10.1016/S0140-6736 (17) 30569-X. PMID: 28402827.

Baker, Tamara A., NiCole T. Buchanan, Chivon A. Mingo, Rosalyn Roker, Candace S. Brown. "Reconceptualizing Successful Aging Among Black Women and the Relevance of the Strong Black Woman Archetype." *The Gerontologist*, 55, 1 (2015): 51–57. https://doi.org/10.1093/geront/gnu105.

Barak, Katie Sullivan. "Spinsters, old maids, and cat ladies: A case study in containment strategies." PhD diss., Bowling Green State University, 2014, 1–221. https://etd.ohiolink.edu/apexprod/rws_etd/send_file/send?accessi on=bgsu1393246792&disposition=inline.

Barrett, Anne E., and Cheryl Robbins. "The Multiple Sources of Women's Aging Anxiety and Their Relationship With Psychological Distress." *Journal of Aging & Health*, 20, 1 (2008): 32–65. https://doi.org/10.1177/0898264307309932.

Barrett, Jennifer. "Here's One More Way Women Get Shortchanged on Money Matters." *The Daily Beast*, May 16, 2021. https://www.thedailybeast.com/heres-one-more-way-women-get-shortchanged-on-money-matters.

———, *Think Like a Breadwinner: A Wealth-Building Manifesto for Women Who Want to Earn More (and Worry Less)*. New York: G.P. Putnam's Sons, 2021.

Barrie, Thorne. "Girls and Boys Together . . . but Mostly Apart: Gender Arrangements in Elementary Schools." In *Relationships and Development*, edited by Willard Hartup and Rubin Zick, 167–84. New Jersey, Lawrence Erlbaum, 1986.

Bateman, Justine, *Face: One Square Foot of Skin*. New York: Akashic, 2021.

Beau, Elle. "Hot Sex Is Not Just for the Young." *Sensual: An Erotic Life*, December 13, 2020. https://medium.com/sensual-enchantment/hot-sex-is-not-just-for-the-young-fc2ffcec93ba.

Beauvais, Julian. "Golden Girls: 5 Times Dorothy and Blanche Were Closer Than Sisters (& 5 Times They Were At Each Other's Throats)." *Screen Rant*, April 4, 2021. https://screenrant.com/golden-girls-5-times-dorothy-and-blanche-were-closer-than-sisters-5-times-they-were-at-each-others-throats.

Benjamin, Rich. "Op-Ed: The president-elect and his VP both provide great models for matrimony." *Los Angeles Times*, November 15, 2020. https://www.latimes.com/opinion/story/2020-11-15/the-president-elect-and-his-veep.

Bening, Annette. "Acting Is 'A Fabulous Way to Expand Your Own Heart.'" Interview by Terry Gross, *Fresh Air*, NPR, May 10, 2018. Audio, 36:00. http://www.npr./2018/05/10/610014961/annette-bening-acting-is-a-fabulous-way-to-expand-your-own-heart.

Berdychevsky, Liza, and Galit Nimrod, "Sex as Leisure in Later Life: A Netnographic Approach." *Leisure Sciences*, 39:3 (2017): 224–43.

Berkowitz, Gale. "UCLA Study On Friendship Among Women," 2002. http://www.anapsid.org/cnd/gender/tendfend.html.

Bertsche, Rachel. *MWF Seeking BFF: My Yearlong Search for a New Best Friend*. New York: Ballantine Books, 2012.

Bialosky, Jill. "How We Became Strangers" in *The Bitch in the House: 26 Women Tell the Truth About Sex, Solitude, Work, Motherhood, and Marriage*, edited by Cathi Hanauer, 119. New York: William Morrow Paperbacks, 2003.

Bielski, Zosia. "The new reality of dating over 65: Men want to live together; women don't." *The Globe and Mail*, November 26, 2019. https://www.the globeandmail.com/life/relationships/article-women-older-than-65-dont -want-to-live-with-their-partners.

Bindley, Katie. "Gen X Women Succeed at Work, Have Fewer Kids: Study." *HuffPost*, September 13, 2011. https://www.huffpost.com/entry/gen-x -study_n_959256.

Blackstone, Amy. "Grow Old Like 'The Golden Girls.'" *New York Times*, June 7, 2019. https://www.nytimes.com/2019/06/07/opinion/retirement -aging-golden-girls.html.

Bleiweis, Robin. "Quick Facts About the Gender Wage Gap." *Center for American Progress*, March 24, 2020. https://www.americanprogress.org/ issues/women/reports/2020/03/24/482141/quick-facts-gender-wage-gap.

Blevins, Joe. "Read This: How the Golden Girls nurtured its considerable gay following." *AV Club*, March 8, 2016. https://www.avclub.com/read -this-how-the-golden-girls-nurtured-its-considerab-1798244966.

Blieszner, Rosemary, Aaron Ogletree, and Rebecca Adams. "Friendship in Later Life: A Research Agenda." *Innovation in Aging*. 3, 1 (2019): igz005, https://doi.org/10.1093/geroni/igz005.

Boaler, Jo. "Parents' Beliefs about Math Change Their Children's Achieve-ment." *YouCubed*. https://www.youcubed.org/resources/parents-beliefs -math-change-childrens-achievement.

Bowen, Sesali, *Notes From a Trap Feminist: A Manifesto for the Bad Bitch Gen-eration*. New York: Amistad, 2021.

———. "What Women Who Criticize Plastic Surgery Don't See." *New York Times*, March 4, 2020. https://www.nytimes.com/2020/03/04/opinion/ black-women-plastic-surgery-natural.html.

Bowman, Cynthia Grant. "Living Apart Together as a 'Family Form' Among Persons of Retirement Age: The Appropriate Family Law Re-sponse." *Family Law Quarterly* 52, 1 (2018): 1–25.

Brady, Lois Smith. "The Writer Anne Lamott Gets to the Happily-Ever-After Part." *New York Times*, April 26, 2019. https://www.nytimes .com/2019/04/26/fashion/weddings/the-final-chapters-of-anne-lamotts -life-now-include-a-soul-mate.html.

Braff, Danielle. "From Best Friends to Platonic Spouses." *New York Times*, May 1, 2021. *NYTimes.com*. https://www.nytimes.com/2021/05/01/fashion/ weddings/from-best-friends-to-platonic-spouses.html.

Brailey, Carla D., and Brittany C. Slatton. "Women, Work, and Inequality in the U.S.: Revisiting the 'Second-Shift.'" *The Journal of Sociology and Social Work* 7 (2019): 1–6.

Brake, Elizabeth. *Minimizing Marriage: Marriage, Morality, and the Law.* England: Oxford University Press, 2012.

———. "Recognizing Care: The Case for Friendship and Polyamory." *Splace Journal,* 1 (2013). https://slace.syr.edu/issue-1-2013-14-on-equality/recognizing-care-the-case-for-friendship-and-polyamory.

Bretschneider, Judy G., and Norma L. McCoy. "Sexual interest and behavior in healthy 80- to 102-year-olds." *Archives of Sexual Behavior* 17, (1988): 109–29. https://doi.org/10.1007/BF01542662.

Bridges, Tristan, and Melody L. Boyd. "On Straight Men's Marriageability Across the Class Divide." *Feminist Reflections,* December 7, 2016. https://thesocietypages.org/feminist/2016/12/07/on-straight-mens-marriageability-across-the-class-divide.

Brinig, Margaret F., and Douglas W. Allen. "'These boots are made for walking': Why most divorce filers are women." *American Law and Economics Review* 2, 1 (January 2000): 126–69. https://doi.org/10.1093/aler/2.1.126.

Brodeur, Nicole. "'Love and Trouble': Claire Dederer's midlife take on sex and self-perception." *The Seattle Times,* May 5, 2021. https://www.seattletimes.com/entertainment/books/why-was-i-a-gigantic-slut-claire-dederers-midlife-take-on-love-sex-and-trouble.

Brooks, Abigail T. "Opting In or Opting Out?: North American Women Share Strategies for Aging Successfully with (and Without) Cosmetic Intervention" in *Successful Aging as a Contemporary Obsession: Global Perspectives,* edited by Sarah Lamb, New Jersey: Rutgers University Press, 2017.

Brooks, Kim, and The Cut, "The changing reasons why women cheat on their husbands." *CNN,* March 13, 2018. https://www.cnn.com/2017/10/05/health/why-women-cheat-partner/index.html.

Brooks, Kim. "The Emancipation of the MILF." *The Cut,* May 18, 2017. https://www.thecut.com/2017/05/female-sexuality-desire-what-happens-as-women-age.html.

———. "Married With Benefits." *Chicago Magazine,* April 23, 2019. https://www.chicagomag.com/Chicago-Magazine/May-2019/Married-With-Benefits.

———. "Who So Many Women Cheat on Their Husbands." *The Cut,* September 21, 2017. https://www.thecut.com/2017/09/why-women-cheat-esther-perel-state-of-affairs.html.

Brown, Susan L., and I-Fen Lin. "The Gray Divorce Revolution: Rising Divorce Among Middle-Aged and Older Adults, 1990–2010." *The Journals of Gerontology: Series B,* 67, 6 (November 2012): 731–41. https://doi.org/10.1093/geronb/gbs089.

Bruni Lopez y Royo, Alessandra. "Modeling as an Older Woman: Exploitation or Subversion?," *Age Culture Humanities,* 2 (2015): 295–308. https://ageculturehumanities.org/WP/modeling-as-an-older-woman-exploitation-or-subversion.

Bui, Quoctrung, and Claire Cain Miller. "The Age That Women Have Babies: How a Gap Divides America." *New York Times*. August 24, 2018. https://www.nytimes.com/interactive/2018/08/04/upshot/up-birth-age-gap.html.

Burgmann, Jennifer. "Why I'm Afraid of Aging With a Disability." *The Mighty*, February 17, 2020. https://www.yahoo.com/now/why-im-afraid-aging-disability-224042506.html.

Busch, Akiko, "The Invisibility of Older Women." *The Atlantic*. February 27, 2019. https://www.theatlantic.com/entertainment/archive/2019/02/akiko-busch-mrs-dalloway-shows-aging-has-benefits/583480.

Butrica, Barbara A., and Karen E. Smith. "The Retirement Prospects of Divorced Women." *Social Security Bulletin*, 72, 1 (2012): 11–22. https://www.ssa.gov/policy/docs/ssb/v72n1/v72n1p11.html.

Calasanti, Toni, and King, Neal. "Successful Aging, Ageism, and the Maintenance of Age and Gender Relations" in *Successful Aging as a Contemporary Obsession: Global Perspectives*, edited by Sarah Lamb, 27–40. New Jersey: Rutgers University Press, 2017.

Caldwell, Hilary, and John de Wit, "Women's experiences buying sex in Australia—Egalitarian power moves." *Sexualities* 24, no. 4 (June 2021): 549–73. https://doi.org/10.1177/1363460719896972.

Calhoun, Ada, *Wedding Toasts I'll Never Give*. First Edition. New York: W. W. Norton Company, 2017.

———. *Why We Can't Sleep: Women's New Midlife Crisis*. New York: Grove Paperback, 2021.

Cardos, Nicole. "Why One Sociologist Says It's Time for Black Women to Date White Men." *WTTW*, April 17, 2019. https://news.wttw.com/2019/04/17/sociologist-cheryl-judice-interracial-relationships.

Carstensen, Laura. *A Long Bright Future: Happiness, Health, and Financial Security in an Age of Increased Longevity*. New York: Harmony, 2009.

Cartner-Morley, Jess. "Shades of 50: How the midlife woman went from invisible to the main event." *The Guardian*. March 21, 2020. https://www.theguardian.com/fashion/2020/mar/21/shades-of-50-how-the-midlife-woman-went-from-invisible-to-the-main-event.

"The Case for An Older Woman." *OkCupid*, February 16, 2010. https://theblog.okcupid.com/the-case-for-an-older-woman-99d8cabacdf5.

Cath, Danielle C., Krystal Nizar, Dorret Boomsma, Carol A. Mathews. "Age-Specific Prevalence of Hoarding and Obsessive Compulsive Disorder: A Population-Based Study." *The American Journal of Geriatric Psychiatry*, 25, 3 (2017): 245–55. https://doi.org/10.1016/j.jagp.2016.11.006.

Centre for Ageing Better. "Dominant narratives on ageing." Accessed March 15, 2021, https://www.ageing-better.org.uk/sites/default/files/2020-11/dominant-narratives-ageing-full-report.pdf.

Centers for Disease and Control, "Disability Impacts All of Us." September 20, 2020. https://www.cdc.gov/ncbddd/disabilityandhealth/infographic-disability-impacts-all.html.

Centers for Disease Control and Prevention, "Atlas Plus: HIV, Hepatitis, STD, TB, Social Determines of Health Data." 2018. https://gis.cdc.gov/grasp/nchhstpatlas/charts.html.

Centers for Disease Control and Prevention, "Sexually Transmitted Disease Surveillance 2019: Reported STDs in the U.S. reach all-time high for 6th consecutive year." April 13, 2021. https://www.cdc.gov/std/statistics/2019/default.htm.

Chan, Shirley, Alyssa Gomes, and Rama Shankar Singh. "Is menopause still evolving? Evidence from a longitudinal study of multiethnic populations and its relevance to women's health." *BMC Women's Health* 20, 74 (2020). https://doi.org/10.1186/s12905-020-00932-8.

Chella, Cailley. "Paulina Porizkova, 54, says she shares 'the truth' about being an older woman to help others: 'We are all in the same frickin' boat!'" *The Daily Mail.* July 18, 2019. https://www.dailymail.co.uk/tvshowbiz/article-7263077/Paulina-Porizkova-54-says-shares-truth-older-woman-help-others.html.

Chemaly, Soraya. "Coronavirus could hurt women the most. Here's how to prevent a patriarchal pandemic." *Think,* April 20, 2020. https://www.nbcnews.com/think/opinion/coronavirus-could-hurt-women-most-here-s-how-prevent-patriarchal-ncna1186581.

Cheung, Elaine O., Wendi L. Gardner, and Jason F. Anderson. "Emotionships: Examining People's Emotion-Regulation Relationships and Their Consequences for Well-Being." *Social Psychological and Personality Science* 6, 4 (May 2015): 407–14. https://doi.org/10.1177/1948550614564223.

"Childless women more likely to begin menopause early, study finds." *National Child Development Study,* January 25, 2017. https://ncds.info/childless-women-more-likely-to-begin-menopause-early-study-finds.

Chinnappan, Shivani. "Long COVID: The Impact on Women and Ongoing Research." *Society for Women's Health Research,* March 18, 2002. https://swhr.org/long-covid-the-impact-on-women-and-ongoing-research.

Chivers, Sally. "How we rely on older adults, especially during the coronavirus pandemic." *The Conversation,* July 30, 2020. https://theconversation.com/how-we-rely-on-older-adults-especially-during-the-coronavirus-pandemic-143346.

Chrisler, Joan. "Teaching Taboo Topics: Menstruation, Menopause, and the Psychology of Women." *Psychology of Women Quarterly,* 37 (2013): 128–32. 10.1177/0361684312471326.

Chrisler, Joan, Angela Barney, and Brigida Palatino. "Ageism Can be Hazardous to Women's Health: Ageism, Sexism, and Stereotypes of Older Women in the Healthcare System." *Journal of Social Issues* 72 (2016): 86–104. 10.1111/josi.12157.

Cleghorn, Elinor. *Unwell Women: Misdiagnosis and Myth in a Man-Made World.* New York: Dutton, 2021.

Clements, Erin. "'Golden Girls producer Tony Thomas on show's popularity: 'What we built was a family.'" *Today,* June 6, 2019. https://www.today.com/popculture/golden-girls-producer-tony-thomas-show-s-popularity-what-we-t154185.

Cochrane, Kira. "Why it's never too late to be a lesbian." *The Guardian,* July 22, 2010. https://www.theguardian.com/lifeandstyle/2010/jul/22/late-blooming-lesbians-women-sexuality.

Cohen, Patricia. *In Our Prime: The Invention of Middle Age.* New York: Scribner, 2012.

Cohen, Philip. "Marriage rates among people with disabilities (save the data edition)." *The Society Pages,* November 11, 2014. https://thesocietypages.org/ccf/2014/11/24/marriage-rates-among-people-with-disabilities-save-the-data-edition.

Cohen, Rhaina. "What If Friendship, Not Marriage, Was at the Center of Life?" *The Atlantic,* October 20, 2020. https://www.theatlantic.com/family/archive/2020/10/people-who-prioritize-friendship-over-romance/616779.

Cohn, D'Vera, Gretchen Livingston, and Wendy Wang. "After Decades of Decline, A Rise in Stay-at-Home Mothers." *Pew Research Center,* April 8, 2014. https://www.pewresearch.org/social-trends/2014/04/08/after-decades-of-decline-a-rise-in-stay-at-home-mothers.

Cohn, D'Vera, and Jeffrey S. Passel. "A record 64 million Americans live in multigenerational households." *Pew Research Center,* April 5, 2018. https://www.pewresearch.org/fact-tank/2018/04/05/a-record-64-million-americans-live-in-multigenerational-households.

Coleman, Joshua. "A Shift in American Family Values." *The Atlantic,* January 10, 2021. https://www.theatlantic.com/family/archive/2021/01/why-parents-and-kids-get-estranged/617612.

Coombs, Robert H. "Marital Status and Personal Well-Being: A Literature Review." *Family Relations* 40, 1 (1991): 97–102. https://doi.org/10.2307/585665.

Coontz, Stephanie. "How to Make Your Marriage Gayer." *New York Times,* February 13, 2020. https://www.nytimes.com/2020/02/13/opinion/sunday/marriage-housework-gender-happiness.html.

Copaken, Deborah. "The Case of the Vanishing Woman." *Next Avenue.* January 7, 2015. https://www.nextavenue.org/case-vanishing-woman.

Coren, Michael J. "Are millennials really giving up on children over climate change?" *Quartz.* December 3, 2020. https://qz.com/1940690/are-millennials-really-giving-up-on-children-over-climate-change.

Coupland, Justine, and Gwyn, Richard, editors, *Discourse, the Body, and Identity,* New York: Palgrave Macmillan, 2003.

Crowley, Jocelyn Elise. "Baby boomers are divorcing for surprisingly old-fashioned reasons." *Aeon,* May 7, 2018. https://aeon.co/ideas/baby-boomers-are-divorcing-for-surprisingly-old-fashioned-reasons.

Cuffari, Elena Clare. "Friendless Women and the Myth of Male Nonage: Why We Need a Better Science of Love and Sex" in *New Philosophies of*

Sex and Love: Thinking Through Desire, edited by Sarah LaChance Adams, Christopher M. Davidson, Caroline R. Lundquist 105–106, New York: Rowman & Littlefield Publishers, 2016.

Cundall, Amanda, and Kun Guo. "Women gaze behaviour in assessing female bodies: The effects of clothing, body size, own body composition and body satisfaction." *Psychological Research* 81 (2017): 1–12. https://doi.org/10.1007/s00426-015-0726-1.

Cunha, Darlena. "I'm One of the 56% of American Mothers Who 'Prefer' to Stay Home." *Time,* October 9, 2015. https://time.com/4068559/gallup-poll-stay-at-home-mothers.

Davis, Lisa Selin. "Amid an epidemic of loneliness, some friendships grow stronger." *CNN,* October 8, 2020. https://www.cnn.com/2020/10/05/health/fewer-but-stronger-friendships-wellness/index.html.

———. "Why Modern Medicine Keeps Overlooking Menopause." *New York Times,* April 6, 2021. https://www.nytimes.com/2021/04/06/us/menopause-perimenopause-symptoms.html.

Day, Jody. "I'm Losing My Shame." *The Age Buster,* November 20, 2020. https://www.theagebuster.com/blog-page/2020/11/20/im-losing-my-shame.

DeMaio, Krista Bennett, and Erin Stovall. "Beauty Brands Are Catering to Women Over 50—Finally." *Oprah Daily,* February 19, 2020. https://www.oprahmag.com/beauty/a30980789/beauty-brands-women-over-50/.

Dennerstein, Lorraine, Philippe Lehert, and Henry Burger. "The relative effects of hormones and relationship factors on sexual function of women through the natural menopausal transition." *Reproductive endocrinology* 84, 1, (2005): 174–80. https://doi.org/10.1016/j.fertnstert.2005.01.119.

DePaulo, Bella. *How We Live Now: Redefining Home and Family in the 21st Century.* Oregon: Atria Books/Beyond Words, 2015.

———. "If you aren't in a relationship, who is your 'person?'" *Washington Post,* April 4, 2018. https://www.washingtonpost.com/news/soloish/wp/2018/04/04/if-youre-single-who-is-your-person.

Deresiewicz, William. "A Man. A Woman. Just Friends?" *New York Times,* April 8, 2012. https://www.nytimes.com/2012/04/08/opinion/sunday/a-man-a-woman-just-friends.html.

DeSantis, Rachel, and Charlotte Triggs. "Sheryl Sandberg Is Engaged to Tom Bernthal After Being Set Up by Her Late Husband's Brother." *People,* February 3, 2020. https://people.com/human-interest/sheryl-sandberg-engaged-tom-bernthal.

Diamond, S. J. "Sequel / 'Phenomenon' Authors." *Los Angeles Times.* February 1, 1993. https://www.latimes.com/archives/la-xpm-1993-02-01-vw-992-story.html.

Dolan, Leah. "Teens are worried about wrinkles. Here's how Gen Z is helping to fuel a beauty boom." *CNN,* May 6, 2021. https://www.cnn.com/style/article/anti-aging-trend-teens/index.html.

Donizzetti, Anna Rosa. "Ageism in an Aging Society: The Role of Knowledge, Anxiety about Aging, and Stereotypes in Young People and Adults." *International journal of environmental research and public health*, 16, 8, (2019): 1329. https://doi.org/10.3390/ijerph16081329.

Druckerman, Pamela. *There Are No Grown-Ups: A Midlife Coming-of-Age Story*. New York: Penguin Press, 2018.

Drummond, J. D., Shari Brotman, Marjorie Silverman, Tamara Sussman, Pam Orzeck, Lucy Barylak, and Isabelle Wallach. "The Impact of Caregiving: Older Women's Experiences of Sexuality and Intimacy." *Affilia*: Journal of Women & Social Work, 28, 4 (2013): 415–28. https://doi.org/10.1177/0886109913504154.

Dumont, Muriel, Marie Sarlet, and Benoit Dardenne. "Be Too Kind to a Woman, She'll Feel Incompetent: Benevolent Sexism Shifts Self-construal and Autobiographical Memories Toward Incompetence." *Sex Roles* 62 (2020): 545–53. 10.1007/s11199-008-9582-4.

Dunsmuir, Lindsay. "Many Americans have no friends of another race: Poll." *Reuters*, August 7, 2013. https://www.reuters.com/article/us-usa-poll-race/many-americans-have-no-friends-of-another-race-poll-idUS BRE97704320130808.

Edwards, Clayton. "'The Golden Girls': Who Was the Youngest Actress on the Show?" *Outsider*, April 1, 2021. https://outsider.com/news/entertainment/golden-girls-who-was-youngest-actress-on-show.

Ellin, Abby. "New Women's Groups Focus on Generational Mix." *New York Times*, November 10, 2018. https://www.nytimes.com/2018/11/10/style/intergenerational-womens-groups.html?

Engeln, Renee. *Beauty Sick: How the Cultural Obsession with Appearance Hurts Girls and Women*. New York: HarperCollins Publishers, 2017.

England, Paula, and Elizabeth Aura McClintock. "The Gendered Double Standard of Aging in US Marriage Markets." *Population and Development Review*, 35(4) (2009): 797–816. https://doi.org/10.1111/j.1728-4457.2009.00309.x.

Ermer, Ashley E., Dikla Segel-Karpas, and Jacquelyn J Benson. "Loneliness trajectories and correlates of social connections among older adult married couples." *JFP: Journal of the Division of Family Psychology of the American Psychological Association (Division 43)*, 34, 8, (2020): 1014–24. https://doi.org/10.1037/fam0000652.

Ermer, Ashley E., and Kristin N. Matera. "Older women's friendships: Illuminating the role of marital histories in how older women navigate friendships and caregiving for friends." *Journal of Women & Aging*, 33, 2 (2021): 214–29. https://doi.org/10.1080/08952841.2020.1860632.

Eugenie Allen. "Get Back to Work." Review of *The Feminine Mistake*, by Leslie Bennetts. *New York Times*, May 6, 2007. https://www.nytimes.com/2007/05/06/books/review/Allen.t.html.

Evans, Jane. The Uninvisibility Project. Accessed June 2, 2021. https://www.uninvisibility.com.

Exploring Your Mind, "Sawubona: An African Trib's Beautiful Greeting." October 1, 2018. https://exploringyourmind.com/sawubona-african-tribe -greeting.

Fabbre, Vanessa. "Gender Transitions in Later Life: The Significance of Time in Queer Aging." *Journal of Gerontological Social Work*, 57 (2–4) (2014): 161–75. https://doi.org/10.1080/01634372.2013.855287.

Feldman, H. A., I. Goldstein, D. G. Hatzichristou, R. J. Krane, and J. B. McKinlay. "Impotence and its medical and psychosocial correlates: Results of the Massachusetts Male Aging Study." *Journal of Urology*, 151, 1 (1994): 54–61.

Felmlee, Diane, and Anna Muraco. "Gender and Friendship Norms Among Older Adults," *Research on Aging*, 31, 3 (2009): 318–44. https://doi .org/10.1177/0164027508330719.

Fileborn, Bianca, Rachel Thorpe, Gail Hawkes, Victor Minichiello, Marian Pitts, and Tinashe Dune. "Sex, desire and pleasure: Considering the experiences of older Australian women." *Sexual and relationship therapy: Journal of the British Association for Sexual and Relationship Therapy*, 30, 1 (2015). 117–30. https://doi.org/10.1080/14681994.2014.936722.

Finkel, Eli J. *The All-Or-Nothing Marriage: How the Best Marriages Work*. New York: Dutton, 2019.

"For women, sexuality changes with age but doesn't disappear." *Harvard Health Publishing*, July 21, 2019. https://www.health.harvard.edu/blog/for -women-sexuality-changes-with-age-but-doesnt-disappear-201402137035.

Foreman, Amanda. "Why Footbinding Persisted in China for a Millennium." *Smithsonian Magazine*, February 2015. https://www.smithsonianmag.com/ history/why-footbinding-persisted-china-millennium-180953971.

Fox, Michelle. "How women can take control of their money and grow their wealth," *CNBC*, September 6, 2019. https://www.cnbc.com/2019/09/06/ how-women-can-take-control-of-their-money-and-grow-their-wealth .html.

Frankel, Valerie. "You gotta have friends!," *Self*, October 7, 2009. https:// www.self.com/story/how-many-friends-do-you-need.

Frederick, David A., H. Kate St. John, Justin R. Garcia, and Elisabeth A. Lloyd. "Differences in Orgasm Frequency Among Gay, Lesbian, Bisexual, and Heterosexual Men and Women in a U.S. National Sample." *Archives of sexual behavior*, 47 (1) (2018): 273–88. https://doi.org/10.1007/s10508-017 -0939-z.

Fristoe, Kerry. "Robin Hauser Wants Women to Get Savvy About Their Personal Finances." *Lioness Magazine*, March 31, 2021. https://lionessmagazine .com/robin-hauser-wants-women-to-get-savvy-about-their-personal -financess.

Fulton, Rick. "Susan Boyle's life story to be turned into movie with Meryl Streep." *Daily Record*, November 21, 2019. https://www.dailyrecord.co .uk/news/scottish-news/movie-scots-superstar-susan-boyles-20925022.

Funderburg, Lise. "The Two Friends Every Woman Needs." *Good House-keeping*, January 25, 2012. https://www.goodhousekeeping.com/life/inspi rational-stories/a19612/long-lasting-friendships.

Gallagher, James. "Fertility rate: 'Jaw-dropping' global crash in children being born," *BBC*, July 15, 2020. https://www.bbc.com/news/health-53409521.

Garber, Megan. "When Newsweek 'Struck Terror in the Hearts of Single Women." *The Atlantic*, June 2016. https://www.theatlantic.com/entertain ment/archive/2016/06/more-likely-to-be-killed-by-a-terrorist-than-to-get -married/485171.

Garner, J. Dianne. "Feminism and feminist gerontology." *Journal of Women & Aging*, 11 (1999): 3–12. https://doi.org/10.1300/J074v11n02_02.

Geena Davis Institute on Gender in Media. "TENA partners with the Geena Davis Institute on Gender in Media to launch new 'Ageless Test' to tackle ageism in media." October 9, 2020. https://seejane.org/gender-in-media -news-release/tena-partners-with-the-geena-davis-institute-on-gender -in-media-to-launch-new-ageless-test-to-tackle-ageism-in-media.

"Gender and Stress," *American Psychological Association*, 2012, https://www .apa.org/news/press/releases/stress/2010/gender-stress.

Geronimus, Arline T., Margaret T. Hicken, Jay A. Pearson, Sarah J. Seashols, Kelly L. Brown, and Tracey Dawson Cruz. "Do US Black Women Experience Stress-Related Accelerated Biological Aging?: A Novel Theory and First Population-Based Test of Black-White Differences in Telomere Length." *Human Nature*, 21, 1 (2010): 19–38. https://doi.org/10.1007/ s12110-010-9078-0.

Gilbert, Fritz. "What Baby Boomer Women Need to Know About Their Finances." *The Retirement Manifesto*, July 4, 2017. https://www.theretire mentmanifesto.com/what-baby-boomer-women-need-to-know-about -their-finances.

Gillan, Tamara. "Why are the majority of women struggling with self-esteem issues?" *StartUps Magazine*. https://startupsmagazine.co.uk/article -why-are-majority-women-struggling-self-esteem-issues.

Glennon, Francis. "Meaty Meadisms About America." *Life*, September 14, 1959, 47, No. 11. Google Books.

Glynn, Sarah Jane. "Breadwinning Mothers Continue to Be the U.S. Norm." *Center for American Progress*, May 10, 2019. https://www.american progress.org/issues/women/reports/2019/05/10/469739/breadwinning -mothers-continue-u-s-norm.

Gold, Michael. "Helping Women Overcome Society's Outdated Messages on Money." *New York Times*, June 17, 2019. https://www.nytimes.com/ 2019/06/17/business/sallie-krawcheck-stephanie-cohen-new-rules.html.

Gordon, Emily V. "Why Women Compete With Each Other." *New York Times*, October 31, 2015. https://www.nytimes.com/2015/11/01/opinion/ sunday/why-women-compete-with-each-other.html.

Gottberg, Kathy. "Rightsizing Your Finances—A SMART Way to Manage Money." *SMART Living*, 365, https://www.smartliving365.com/rightsizing -your-finances-a-smart-way-to-manage-money.

Goudarzi, Sara. "Men as Addicted to Shopping as Women." *Live Science,* September 30, 2006. https://www.livescience.com/1036-men-addicted -shopping-women.html.

Graham, Cynthia A., C. H. Mercer, C. Tanton, K. G. Jones, A. M. Johnson, K. Wellings, and K. R. Mitchell. "What factors are associated with reporting lacking interest in sex and how do these vary by gender? Findings from the third British national survey of sexual attitudes and lifestyles," *BMJ Open*, vol. 7, 9 e016942. (September 13, 2017), doi:10.1136/bmjopen -2017-016942.

Griffin, Eden M., and Karen L. Fingerman, "Online Dating Profile Content of Older Adults Seeking Same- and Cross-Sex Relationships." *Journal of GLBT Family Studies,* 14 (2017): 446–66. https://doi.org/10.1080/15504 28X.2017.1393362.

Gullette, Margaret Morganroth. *Declining to Decline: Cultural Combat and the Politics of the Midlife.* Virginia: University Press of Virginia Charlottesville, 1997.

Gunter, Jen. *The Menopause Manifesto: Own Your Health with Facts and Feminism.* New York: Citadel Press, 2021.

———. "When the Cause of a Sexless Relationship Is—Surprise!— the Man." *New York Times,* March 10, 2018. https://www.nytimes .com/2018/03/10/style/sexless-relationships-men-low-libido.html.

———. "Women Can Have a Better Menopause. Here's How." *New York Times,* May 25, 2021. https://www.nytimes.com/2021/05/25/opinion/ feminist-menopause.html.

Gupta, Swati, and Sugam Pokharel. "Indian woman gives birth to twins at age of 73." *CNN.* September 6, 2019. https://www.cnn.com/2019/09/06/ health/india-woman-73-gives-birth-scli-intl.

Hafford-Letchfield, Trish, N. Lambert, E. Long, and D. Brady. "Going Solo: Findings from a survey of women ageing without a partner and who do not have children." *Journal of Women & Aging,* 29, 4 (2017): 321–33. doi:10 .1080/08952841.2016.1187544.

Hale, Julie. "Betsey Prioleau: A bewitching new book offers lessons in love." *BookPage,* December 2003. https://bookpage.com/interviews/8231-betsey -prioleau-history#.YEw_-h2IYkg.

Hall, Marcella Runell, and Kersha Smith, editors, *UnCommon Bonds: Women Reflect on Race and Friendship.* New Edition. Switzerland: Peter Lang Inc., International Academic Publishers, 2018.

Halstead, Richard. "Buck Institute in Novato expands reproduction research." *Marin Independent Journal.* September 30, 2019. https://www .marinij.com/2019/09/30/buck-institute-in-novato-expands-reproduction -research.

Hannon, Kerry. "Opinion: This is why so many women face poverty in their old age." *MarketWatch*, September 29, 2020. https://www.market watch.com/story/this-is-why-so-many-women-face-poverty-in-their-old -age-2020-09-29.

Hamilton, Brady E., Joyce A. Martin, and Michelle J. K. Osterman, M.H.S. "Births: Provisional Data for 2019." *Division of Vital Statistics, National Center for Health Statistics*, May 2020. https://www.cdc.gov/nchs/data/ vsrr/vsrr-8-508.pdf.

Hanson, Kait. "New Hampshire woman gives birth at 57." *Today*. March 24, 2021. https://www.today.com/parents/new-hampshire-woman-gives -birth-57-t212902.

Hardy, Sarah. "Fashion vs Naturism: Amelia Allen Launches Naked Britain Photography Book via Kehrer Verlag." *FMS*, November 13, 2017. https:// fms-mag.com/fashion-vs-naturism-amelia-allen-launches-naked-britain -photography-book-via-kehrer-verlag.

Harris, Kandace L. "'Follow Me on Instagram': 'Best Self' Identity Con-struction and Gaze through Hashtag Activism and Selfie Self-Love." *In Women of Color and Social Media: Multitasking Blogs, Timelines, Feeds, and Community*, edited by S. M. Brown Givens and K. Edwards Tassie, 133. Maryland: Lexington Books, 2015.

Heggeness, Misty L. "The Up Side of Divorce?: When Laws Make Divorce Easier, Research Shows Women Benefit, Outcomes Improve." *U.S. Cen-sus Bureau*, December 18, 2019. https://www.census.gov/library/stories/ 2019/12/the-upside-of-divorce.html.

Henig, Robin Marantz. "The Last Day of Her Life." *New York Times*, May 14, 2015. https://www.nytimes.com/2015/05/17/magazine/the-last -day-of-her-life.html.

Herrick, Harry, Karen J. Luken, and Pam Dickens. "Women with disabilities and heart disease (North Carolina BRFSS Surveillance Update No. 5)." Raleigh, NC: State Center for Health Statistics, North Carolina Division of Public Health, 2011. https://fpg.unc.edu/sites/fpg.unc.edu/files/resources/ reports-and-policy-briefs/SurveillanceUpdate5_WomenWithDisabilities AndHeartDisease_2011.pdf.

Herzig, Rebecca, *Plucked: A History of Hair Removal*. New York: New York Unversity Press, 2015.

Hill, Faith. "What It's Like to Date After Middle Age." *The Atlantic*, Janu-ary 8, 2020. https://www.theatlantic.com/family/archive/2020/01/dating -after-middle-age-older/604588/.

Hinchliff, Sharron. "When it comes to older people and sex, doctors put their heads in the sand." *The Conversation*, June 19, 2015. https://thecon versation.com/when-it-comes-to-older-people-and-sex-doctors-put-their -heads-in-the-sand-43556.

Hinsliff, Gaby. "'A weird liberation': Why women are exposing the wild truth about midlife and menopause." *The Guardian*, September 22, 2020.

https://www.theguardian.com/lifeandstyle/2020/sep/22/weird-liberation
-women-wild-truth-midlife-menopause.

Hiroshima University. "Some women's retirement plan: Rely on Prince Charming." *ScienceDaily*, www.sciencedaily.com/releases/2016/06/1606 22102127.htm.

Hirsch, Marianne. "Women's Ways of Aging." *Public Books*. June 6, 2020. https://www.publicbooks.org/womens-ways-of-aging.

Hofmeier, Sara M., Cristin D. Runfola, Margarita Sala, Danielle A. Gagne, Kimberly A. Brownley, and Cynthia M. Bulik. "Body image, aging, and identity in women over 50: The Gender and Body Image (GABI) study." *Journal of Women & Aging*, 29, 1 (2017): 3–14. https://doi.org/10.1080/0895 2841.2015.1065140.

Holstein, Martha B, and Meredith Minkler. "Self, Society, and the 'New Gerontology.'" *The Gerontologist*, 43, 6 (December 2003): 787–96. https://doi.org/10.1093/geront/43.6.787.

Howley, Elaine K. "What to Know About Rising STD Rates Among Seniors." *U.S. News*, December 10, 2018. https://health.usnews.com/health -care/patient-advice/articles/2018-12-10/what-to-know-about-rising-std -rates-among-seniors.

Hubbard, Leigh Ann. "Martha Holstein: Feminism and the Future of Aging." *Silver Century Foundation*, March 8, 2018. https://www.silvercentury .org/2018/03/martha-holstein-feminism-and-the-future-of-aging.

Hunt, Katie. "Work, not sex? The real reason Chinese women bound their feet." *CNN*.

Institute of Medicine (U.S.) Committee on Lesbian, Gay, Bisexual, and Transgender Health Issues and Research Gaps and Opportunities. "Later Adulthood," in *The Health of Lesbian, Gay, Bisexual, and Transgender People: Building a Foundation for Better Understanding* (Washington, D.C.: National Academies Press, 2011). https://www.ncbi.nlm.nih.gov/books/NBK64800.

Jean-Philippe, McKenzie. "How Oprah and Gayle's 45-Year Friendship Began—and Why It's Lasted." *Oprah Daily*, March 4, 2021. https://www .oprahdaily.com/life/relationships-love/a26965035/oprah-and-gayle -friendship.

Jenkins, Jo Ann. *Disrupt Aging: A Bold New Path to Living Your Best Life at Every Age*. New York: PublicAffairs, 2016.

Kaas, M. J. "Geriatric sexuality breakdown syndrome." *The International Journal of Aging and Human Development*, 13 (1) (1981): 71–77, https://doi .org/10.2190/4A16-06AH-HL5A-WKC3.

Kafer, Alison. *Feminist, Queer, Crip*. Indiana: Indiana University Press, 2013.

Kao, Alina, Y. M. Binik, A. Kapuscinski, and S. Khalife. "Dyspareunia in postmenopausal women: a critical review." *Pain research & management*, 13 (3) (2008): 243–54. https://doi.org/10.1155/2008/269571.

Kaplan, Janice. *The Genius of Women From Overlooked to Changing the World*. New York: Dutton, 2021.

Karbo, Karen. "The Accidental Breadwinner." *New York Times*, December 12, 2008. https://www.nytimes.com/2008/12/14/fashion/14love.html.

———. *Yeah, No. Not Happening: How I Found Happiness Swearing Off Self-Improvement and Saying F*ck It All—and How You Can Too*. New York: Harper Wave, 2020.

Karni, Annie. "Paulina Porizkova taking verbal 'shots.'" *New York Post*. October 17, 2010. https://nypost.com/2010/10/17/paulina-porizkova-taking-verbal-shots.

Karvonen-Gutierrez, Carrie A. "The importance of disability as a health issue for mid-life women." *Women's Midlife Health* 1, 10 (2015). https://doi.org/10.1186/s40695-015-0011-x.

Katz, Stephen, and Barbara Marshall. "New sex for old: Lifestyle, consumerism, and the ethics of aging well." *Journal of Aging Studies*, 17 (2003): 3–16. https://doi.org/10.1016/S0890-4065(02)00086-5.

Kehoe, Monika. "Lesbians over sixty-five: A triply invisible minority." *Journal of Homosexuality*, 12 (2020): 139–52. https://doi.org/10.1300/J082v12n03_12.

Kenen, Regina. "Suddenly Single: A Widow's Challenge." *The Society Pages*, July 5, 2018. https://thesocietypages.org/specials/suddenly-single-a-widows-challenge.

Kermond, Clare. "Older women want sex more, not less," *The Sydney Morning Herald*. February 25, 2015. https://www.smh.com.au/lifestyle/life-and-relationships/older-women-want-sex-more-not-less-20150225-13oafi.html.

Kerwin, Ann Marie. "Cindy Gallop Doesn't Care What You Think." *Ad Age*, August 22, 2016. https://adage.com/article/news/cindi-gallop/305457.

Kiesel, Laura. "Women and pain: Disparities in experience and treatment." *Harvard Health*, October 9, 2017. https://www.health.harvard.edu/blog/women-and-pain-disparities-in-experience-and-treatment-2017100912562.

Kilkenny, Katie. "How Anti-Aging Cosmetics Took Over the Beauty World." *Pacific Standard*, August 30, 2017. https://psmag.com/social-justice/how-anti-aging-cosmetics-took-over-the-beauty-world.

Kingsberg, Sheryl A., and Terri Woodard, "Female sexual dysfunction: Focus on low desire." *Obstetrics and gynecology*, 125(2) (2015): 477–86. https://doi.org/10.1097/AOG.0000000000000620.

Kirkman, Linda. "Relationship diversity and the life span: Rural baby boomers in friend-with-benefits relationships," paper presented at the Let's Talk About Sex Conference, Pullman on the Park, Melbourne, Victoria, Australia (September 9, 2015).

Knight, Rebecca. "Balancing feminism with caring about what I look like." *Motherwell*, May 13, 2020. https://motherwellmag.com/2020/05/13/balancing-feminism-with-caring-about-what-i-look-like.

Ko, Ahro, C. M. Pick, J. Y. Kwon, M. Barlev, J. A. Krems, M. E. W. Varnum, R. Neel, M. Peysha, W. Boonyasiriwat, and E. Brandstätter. "Family Matters: Rethinking the Psychology of Human Social Motivation." *Perspectives on Psychological Science* 15, 1 (January 2020): 173–201. https://doi .org/10.1177/1745691619872986.

Laceulle, Hanne. *Aging and Self-Realization: Cultural Narratives about Later Life,* Bielefeld: Transcript Verlag, 2018.

Laganà, Luciana, T. White, D. E. Bruzzone, and C. E. Bruzzone. "Exploring the Sexuality of African American Older Women." *British journal of medicine and medical research,* 4(5), (2013): 1129–1148. https://doi.org/10.9734/ BJMMR/2014/5491.

Laganà, Luciana, and Michelle Maciel. "Sexual desire among Mexican-American older women: A qualitative study." *Culture, Health & Sexuality,* 6 (2010): 705–19. https://doi.org/10.1080/13691058.2010.482673.

Lahad, Kinneret, *A Table for One: A Critical Reading of Singlehood, Gender and Time.* First Edition. England: Manchester University Press, 2017.

LaMotte, Sandee. "It's a myth that women don't want sex as they age, study finds." *CNN,* September 28, 2020. https://www.cnn.com/2020/09/28/ health/sexual-desire-older-women-study-wellness/index.html.

Landau, Meryl Davids. "Oprah's Top Wellness Tips for 2020 and Beyond." *Everyday Health,* January 14, 2020. https://www.everydayhealth.com/ healthy-living/oprahs-top-wellness-tips.

Larson, Nancy C. "Becoming 'One of the Girls: The Transition to Lesbian in Midlife.'" *Affilia,* 21 (2006): 296–305. https://doi.org/10.1177/ 0886109906288911.

Larson, Vicki. "Marin psychotherapist addresses marriage at midlife in new book." *Marin Independent Journal,* January 22, 2018. https://www.marinij .com/2018/01/22/marin-psychotherapist-addresses-marriage-at-midlife -in-new-book.

———. "Never too late to find love, says Mill Valley's Eve Pell." *The Marin Independent Journal,* January 26, 2015. https://www.marinij.com/2015/01/26/ never-too-late-to-find-love-says-mill-valleys-eve-pell.

———. "You can't avoid divorce, and here's why." *OMG Chronicles,* July 28, 2014. http://omgchronicles.vickilarson.com/2014/07/28/you-cant-avoid -divorce-and-heres-why.

Laumann, Edward O., A. Paik, and R. C. Rosen. "Sexual dysfunction in the United States: Prevalence and predictors." *Journal of the American Medical Association* 281 (6) (1999): 537–44. https://doi.org/10.1001/jama.281.6.537.

Lee, Bruce. "Can Covid-19 Coronavirus Cause Long-Term Erectile Dysfunction? Here Are 2 More Studies," *Forbes,* May 16, 2021. https://www .forbes.com/sites/brucelee/2021/05/16/can-covid-19-coronavirus-cause -long-term-erectile-dysfunction-here-are-2-more-studies.

Lees, Paris. "Emma Watson On Being Happily 'Self-Partnered' At 30." *Vogue,* April 15, 2020. https://www.vogue.co.uk/news/article/emma-watson -on-fame-activism-little-women.

Levanon, Asaf, Paula England, and Paul Allison. "Occupational Feminization and Pay: Assessing Causal Dynamics Using 1950–2000 U.S. Census Data." *Social Forces*, 88, 2 (2009): 865–91. https://doi.org/10.1353/sof.0.0264.

Levinson, Kate. *Emotional Currency: A Woman's Guide to Building a Healthy Relationship With Money*. California: Celestial Arts, 2011.

Levy, Vicki, and Colette Thayer. "The Positive Impact of Intergenerational Friendships." *AARP Research*. https://doi.org/10.26419/res.00314.002.

Liberatore, Paul. "Frances McDormand, Marin's media-shy star, lends support to coastal radio station." *Marin Independent Journal*, December 15, 2014. https://www.marinij.com/2014/12/15/frances-mcdormand-marins-media-shy-star-lends-support-to-coastal-radio-station.

Lin, I-Fen, and Susan L. Brown. "Unmarried Boomers Confront Old Age: A National Portrait." *The Gerontologist*, 52, 2 (April 2012): 153–65. https://doi.org/10.1093/geront/gnr141.

Lövgren, Karin. "The Swedish *tant*: A marker of female aging." *Journal of women & aging*, 25, 2 (2013): 119–37. https://doi.org/10.1080/08952841.2013.732826.

Luetke, Maya, Devon Hensel, Debby Herbenick, and Molly Rosenberg. "Romantic Relationship Conflict Due to the COVID-19 Pandemic and Changes in Intimate and Sexual Behaviors in a Nationally Representative Sample of American Adults." *Journal of Sex & Marital Therapy*, 46:8 (2020) 747–62. https://doi.org/10.1080/0092623X.2020.1810185.

Machin, Anna, and Robin Dunbar. "Sex and Gender as Factors in Romantic Partnerships and Best Friendships." *Journal of Relationships Research* 4 (2013): e8. doi:10.1017/jrr.2013.8.

Maciel, Michelle, and Luciana Laganà. "Older women's sexual desire problems: Biopsychosocial factors impacting them and barriers to their clinical assessment." *BioMed research international*, 107–217 (2014). https://doi.org/10.1155/2014/107217.

Maestas, Nicole. "The Return to Work and Women's Employment Decisions." *National Bureau of Economic Research Working Paper*, no. 24429 (March 2018). DOI 10.3386/w24429.

Mandell, Andrea. "Where are real portrayals of women over 50 on screen? New study highlights dearth of leading roles." *USA Today*, October 27, 2020 https://www.usatoday.com/story/entertainment/movies/2020/10/27/women-over-50-losing-out-major-movie-roles-study-finds/6048202002.

Margolies, Lynn. "Competition Among Women: Myth and Reality." *PsychCentral*, May 17, 2016. https://psychcentral.com/lib/competition-among-women-myth-and-reality#3.

Martin, Wednesday. *Untrue: Why Nearly Everything We Believe About Women, Lust, and Infidelity Is Wrong and How the New Science Can Set Us Free*. New York: Little, Brown Spark, 2018.

Mason, C. Nicole, and Alicia Modestino. "'Shecession': The Pandemic's Impact on Women in the Workforce." Interview by Meghna Chakrabarti,

On Point, WBUR, October 22, 2020. Audio, 47:18. https://www.wbur.org/ onpoint/2020/10/22/shecession-the-pandemics-impact-on-women-in-the -workplace.

Matsick, Jes, Mary Kruk, and Britney Wardecker. "Sexual Orientation, Femininity, and Attitudes Toward Menstruation Among Women: Implications for Menopause." *Innovation in Aging*, 4 (Suppl. 1), (2020): 860. https://doi.org/10.1093/geroni/igaa057.3173.

Mattern, Susan. *The Slow Moon Climbs: The Science, History, and Meaning of Menopause*. New Jersey: Princeton University Press, 2019.

McAfee, Tierney. "Antonin Scalia Was with Members of Secretive Society of Elite Hunters When He Died." *People*, February 25, 2016. https:// people.com/sports/antonin-scalia-died-during-getaway-with-members -of-secret-hunting-society.

McCrory, Helen. "How should a woman live her life?," *The Guardian*, April 16, 2021. https://www.theguardian.com/culture/2021/apr/16/helen -mccrory-how-should-a-woman-live-her-life.

McDormand, Frances. "Like Olive Kitteridge, Actress Frances McDormand Was Tired of Supporting Roles." Interview by Melissa Block, *All Things Considered*, NPR, October 31, 2014. Audio, 8:00. https://www.npr .org/2014/10/31/360183633/like-olive-kitteridge-actress-frances-mcdor mand-was-tired-of-supporting-roles.

McGowan, Emma. "The Sex Educator Teaching BDSM to People With Disabilities." *Vice*, December 4, 2017. https://www.vice.com/en/article/ ywnm7v/robin-wilson-beattie-sex-educator-bdsm-disabilities?http:// dx.doi.org/10.1080/01490400.2016.1189368.

McGrath, Laura. "Achieving Visibility: Midlife and Older Women's Literate Practices on Instagram and Blogs," *Literacy in Composition Studies*, 6 (2) (2018). https://licsjournal.org/index.php/LiCS/article/view/728.

McLaughlin, Katie. "5 things women couldn't do in the 1960s." *CNN*, August 25, 2014. https://www.cnn.com/2014/08/07/living/sixties-women -5-things.

McRuer, Robert. *Crip Theory: Cultural Signs of Queerness and Disability*. New York: New York University Press, 2006.

Mead, Rebecca. "The Wives of Others." Review of *The Feminine Mistake*, by Leslie Bennetts. *The New Yorker*, April 16, 2007. https://www.newyorker .com/magazine/2007/04/16/the-wives-of-others.

Medetti, Stefania. "Battle the stigma of old age and keep passion alive." *The Age Buster*, August 28, 2019. https://www.theagebuster.com/blog -page/2019/8/28/battle-the-stigma-of-old-age-and-keep-passion-alive.

Mehta, Clare. "At what age are people usually happiest? New research offers surprising clues." *The Conversation*, April 9, 2021. https://theconversa tion.com/at-what-age-are-people-usually-happiest-new-research-offers -surprising-clues-156906.

Menkin, Josephine A., Theodore F. Robles, Tara L. Gruenewald, Elizabeth K. Tanner, and Teresa E. Seeman. "Positive expectations regarding aging linked to more new friends in later life." *The Journals of Gerontology, Series B: Psychological Sciences and Social Sciences*, 72 (2016): 771–81. https://doi.org/10.1093/geronb/gbv118.

Michon, Kathleen. "How Much Will My Divorce Cost and How Long Will It Take?" *Nolo*, 2019. https://www.nolo.com/legal-encyclopedia/ctp/cost-of-divorce.html.

Mikucka, Małgorzata. "Old-Age Trajectories of Life Satisfaction. Do Singlehood and Childlessness Hurt More When People Get Older?" *Swiss Journal of Sociology* 46, 3 (2020): 397–424. doi: https://doi.org/10.2478/sjs-2020-0020.

Mills, Eleanor. "I was told at Facebook I was middle-aged at 35." *The Daily Mail*, June 16, 2021. https://www.dailymail.co.uk/femail/article-9693729/Sheryl-Sandberg-talks-finding-love-fighting-women-hit-pandemic.html.

Moody, Danielle L. Beatty, Charlotte Brown, Karen A. Matthews, and Joyce T. Bromberger. "Everyday Discrimination Prospectively Predicts Inflammation Across 7 Years in Racially Diverse Midlife Women: Study of Women's Health Across the Nation." *The Journal of Social Issues*, 70, 2 (2014): 298–314. https://doi.org/10.1111/josi.12061.

Moore, Anna. "The sexuality revolution: 'Switching sides' in midlife." *You Magazine*, July 15, 2018. https://www.you.co.uk/changing-sexuality-in-midlife.

Moremen, Robin. "Best Friends: The Role of Confidantes in Older Women's Health." *Journal of Women & Aging*. 20 (2008): 149–67. https://doi.org/10.1300/j074v20n01_11.

Moreno-Domínguez, Silvia, Tania Raposo, and Paz Elipe. "Body Image and Sexual Dissatisfaction: Differences Among Heterosexual, Bisexual, and Lesbian Women." *Frontiers in Psychology*, 10 (2019): 903, https://doi.org/10.3389/fpsyg.2019.00903.

Morris, Charlotte Ann. "The significance of friendship in UK single mothers' intimate lives." *Families, Relationships and Societies*, 8, No. 3 (2019): 427–43. https://doi.org/10.1332/204674318X15262010818254.

Morrissey Stahl, Kate A., J. Gale, D. C. Lewis, and D. Kleiber. "Sex after divorce: Older adult women's reflections." *Journal of Gerontological Social Work*, 61(6) (2018): 659–74. https://doi.org/10.1080/01634372.2018.1486936.

Motley, Apryl. "Single and Loving It." *Sisters from AARP*, November 15, 2019. https://www.sistersletter.com/me-time/single-and-loving-it.

Mottola, Gary. "Gender, Generation and Financial Knowledge: A Six-Year Perspective." *FINRA Investor Education Foundation*, March 2018. https://www.usfinancialcapability.org/downloads/Issue-Brief-Gender-Generation-and-Financial-Knowledge-A-Six-Year-Perspective.pdf.

Mundy, Liza. "The Secret Power of Menopause." *The Atlantic*. October 15, 2019. https://www.theatlantic.com/magazine/archive/2019/10/the-secret-power-of-menopause/596662.

Muraco, Anna, and Karen Fredriksen-Goldsen. "That's what friends do": Informal caregiving for chronically ill midlife and older lesbian, gay, and bisexual adults." *Journal of social and personal relationships*, 28, 8 (2011): 1073–92. https://doi.org/10.1177/0265407511402419.

——. "Turning Points in the Lives of Lesbian and Gay Adults Age 50 and Over." *Advances in Life Course Research*, 30 (2016): 124–32. https://doi.org/10.1016/j.alcr.2016.06.002.

Murray, Sarah Hunter. "Heterosexual Men's Sexual Desire: Supported by, or Deviating from, Traditional Masculinity Norms and Sexual Scripts?" *Sex Roles* 78 (2018): 130–41. https://doi.org/10.1007/s11199-017-0766-7.

Natale, Nicol. "Paulina Porizkova, 55, Says 'Sexy Has No Expiration Date' in Nude Instagram Photo." *Prevention*, February 4, 2021. https://www.prevention.com/life/a35408679/paulina-porizkova-nude-instagram-aging.

Nelson. Shasta. "Friendships Don't Just Happen!: The Guide to Creating a Meaningful Circle of GirlFriends," *Shastanelson.com*. https://www.shastanelson.com/friendships-dont-just-happen.

Nelson-Becker, Holly, and Christina Victor. "Dying alone and lonely dying: Media discourse and pandemic conditions." *Journal of aging studies*, 55, 100878 (2020). https://doi.org/10.1016/j.jaging.2020.100878.

Nikolchev, Alexandra. "A brief history of the birth control pill." *PBS*. May 7, 2010. https://www.pbs.org/wnet/need-to-know/health/a-brief-history-of-the-birth-control-pill/480.

Nimura, Janice P. "Why 'Unwell Women' Have Gone Misdiagnosed for Centuries." Review of *Unwell Women: Misdiagnosis and Myth in a Man-Made World* by Elinor Cleghorn. *New York Times*, June 8, 2021, https://www.nytimes.com/2021/06/08/books/review/unwell-women-elinor-cleghorn.html.

Nordgren, Andie. "The short instructional manifesto for relationship anarchy." *Andie's Log*, July 6, 2012. https://log.andie.se/post/26652940513/the-short-instructional-manifesto-for-relationship.

Nors, Dorthe. "On the Invisibility of Middle-Aged Women." *Literary Hub*. June 22, 2016. https://lithub.com/on-the-invisibility-of-middle-aged-women.

Nosek, Margaret. "The Changing Face of Women with Disabilities: Are We Ready?" *Journal of Women's Health*, 15, 9 (2006): 996–99. https://doi.org/10.1089/jwh.2006.15.996.

Nosek, Margaret, C. Howland, D. H. Rintala, M. E. Young, and G. F. Chanpong. "Study of Women With Physical Disabilities: Final Report." *Sexuality and Disability* 19 (2001): 5–40. 10.1023/A:1010716820677.

Novotney, Amy. "The risks of social isolation." *Monitor on Psychology*, 50, 5 (March 2020): 32. https://www.apa.org/monitor/2019/05/ce-corner-isolation.

Obama, Michelle, *Becoming*, First Edition. New York: Crown, 2018.

Ojewumi, Ola. "I'm Celebrating My Disabled Black Girl Magic Because I'm Done Feeling Invisible." *Self.* November 7, 2018. https://www.self.com/story/disabled-black-girl-magic.

O'Leary, Angie. "Opinion: When women control the wealth, society reaps the benefits." *MarketWatch*, January 4, 2019. https://www.market watch.com/story/when-women-control-the-wealth-society-reaps-the -benefits-2019-01-04.

Oprah.com. "Why Michelle Obama Chose 'Becoming' as the Title of Her Upcoming Memoir." November 12, 2018. https://www.oprah.com/oprahsbookclub/why-michelle-obama-chose-becoming-as-the-title-of -her-memoir.

Oregon State University. "'Aging well' greatly affected by hopes and fears for later life," *ScienceDaily*, January 21, 2021. www.sciencedaily.com/releases /2021/01/210121150929.htm.

Ortman, Jennifer M., Victoria A. Velkoff, and Howard Hogan. "An Aging Nation: The Older Population in the United States." *U.S. Census Bureau*, May 2014, https://www.census.gov/prod/2014pubs/p25-1140.pdf.

Pai, Deanna. "The Gray-Hair Revolution Has Begun." *Glamour*, January 29, 2019. https://www.glamour.com/story/gray-hair-revolution.

Paine, Emily Allen, Debra Umberson, and Corinne Reczek. "Sex in Midlife: Women's Sexual Experiences in Lesbian and Straight Marriages." *Journal of marriage and the family*, 81 (1) (2019): 7–23, https://doi.org/10.1111/jomf.12508.

Pandey, Amarendra, Gurpoonam K. Jatana, and Sidharth Sonthalia. "Cosmeceuticals." In *StatPearls*. Florida: StatPearls Publishing, 2020. https://www.ncbi.nlm.nih.gov/books/NBK544223.

Panhard, Ségolène Isabelle Lozano, and Geneviève Loussouarn. "Greying of the human hair: A worldwide survey, revisiting the '50' rule of thumb." *The British Journal of Dermatology*, 167, 4 (2012): 865–73. https://doi.org/10.1111/j.1365-2133.2012.11095.x.

"Parenting in America." *Pew Research Center*, December 17, 2015. https://www.pewsocialtrends.org/2015/12/17/1-the-american-family-today.

Parish, Sharon J., S. S. Faubion, M. Weinberg, B. Bernick, and S. Mirkin. "The MATE survey: Men's perceptions and attitudes towards menopause and their role in partners' menopausal transition." *Menopause*, 26, 10 (2019): 111016. doi: 10.1097/GME.0000000000001373.

Parker, Kim, Rachel Minkin, and Jesse Bennett. "Economic Fallout From COVID-19 Continues to Hit Lower-Income Americans the Hardest." *Pew Research Center*, September 24, 2020. https://www.pewresearch.org/social-trends/2020/09/24/economic-fallout-from-covid-19-continues-to -hit-lower-income-americans-the-hardest.

Parker, Kim, and Renee Stepler. "Americans see men as the financial providers, even as women's contributions grow." *Pew Research Center*, September 20, 2017. https://www.pewresearch.org/fact-tank/2017/09/20/

americans-see-men-as-the-financial-providers-even-as-womens-contri
butions-grow.

Pasulka, Nicole. "'Cat Knows How to Ignore Men;' A Brief History of Lesbian Cat Ladies." *The Cut*, June 23, 2016. https://www.thecut.com/2016/06/ brief-history-of-lesbian-cat-ladies.html.

Pellot, Emerald. "Meet Astala Vista, the self-proclaimed 'crazy cat lady of drag.'" *In the Know*, January 25, 2021. https://www.intheknow.com/post/ meet-astala-vista-the-self-proclaimed-crazy-cat-lady-of-drag.

Perel, Esther. *The State of Affairs: Rethinking Infidelity*. New York: Harper, 2017.

Petski, Denise. "Emma Thompson Criticizes the 'Utterly Unbalanced' Casting of Older Men With Much Younger Women." *Deadline*, December 25, 2020. https://deadline.com/2020/12/emma-thompson-criticizes-the -utterly-unbalanced-casting-of-older-men-with-much-younger-women -1234661562.

Picheta, Rob. "'Crazy cat ladies' are not a thing, study finds." *CNN*, August 21, 2019. https://www.cnn.com/2019/08/21/health/crazy-cat-lady-study -scli-intl/index.html.

Plagnol, Anke C., and Richard A. Easterlin. "Aspirations, Attainments, and Satisfaction: Life Cycle Differences Between American Women and Men." *Journal of Happiness Studies* 9 (2008): 601–19. https://doi.org/10.1007/ s10902-008-9106-5.

Platt, Christine. "Learning to Love and Let Go: What My Divorce Taught Me About Living With Less." *Real Simple*, June 4, 2021. https://www .realsimple.com/home-organizing/organizing/what-divorce-taught-me -about-decluttering.

———. *The Afrominimalist's Guide to Living with Less*. New York: Tiller Press, 2021.

Plummer, Deborah L., R. T. Stone, L. Powell, and J. Allison. "Patterns of Adult Cross-Racial Friendships: A Context for Understanding Contemporary Race Relations." *Cultural Diversity and Ethnic Minority Psychology*, 22, 4 (2016): 479–94. https://doi.org/10.1037/cdp0000079.

Popova, Maria. "Love Undetectable: Andrew Sullivan on Why Friendship Is a Greater Gift Than Romantic Love." *Brain Pickings*, April 23, 2014. https://www.brainpickings.org/2014/04/23/love-undetectable-andrew -sullivan-friendship.

Poston Jr., Dudley L., and Rogelio Sáenz. "The US white majority will soon disappear forever." *The Conversation*, April 30, 2019. https://theconversa tion.com/the-us-white-majority-will-soon-disappear-forever-115894.

Potârcă, Gina, Melinda Mills, and Wiebke Neberich. "Relationship Preferences Among Gay and Lesbian Online Daters: Individual and Contextual Influences." *Journal of Marriage and Family*, 77, 2 (2015): 523–41. https://doi .org/10.1111/jomf.12177.

"The Prince Charming syndrome." *New Zealand Herald,* April 16, 2004. https://www.nzherald.co.nz/nz/the-prince-charming-syndrome/HCYHB 2HHZBJJ4DVXXZM2L5GTRA.

Prioleau, Betsey. *Seductress: Women Who Ravished the World and Their Lost Art of Love.* New York: Viking, 2003.

Purdie-Vaughns, Valerie, and Richard P. Eibach. "Intersectional Invisibility: The Distinctive Advantages and Disadvantages of Multiple Subordinate-Group Identities." *Sex Roles* 59 (2008): 377–91. https://doi.org/10.1007/s11199-008-9424-4.

Radin, Sara. "Queer Crip Fashion: For Standing Out, Proudly." *Refinery29,* July 24, 2021, https://www.refinery29.com/en-us/2020/07/9921895/queer-crip-fashion-disability-rebirth.

Raley, Kelly, Megan M. Sweeney, and Danielle Wondra. "The Growing Racial and Ethnic Divide in U.S. Marriage Patterns." *The Future of Children,* 25, 2 (2015): 89–109. https://doi.org/10.1353/foc.2015.0014.

Ralston, Jeannie. "Who Are You Calling Invisible?" *Ageist,* January 24, 2019. https://www.weareageist.com/women/who-are-you-calling-invisible.

Rampton, Martha. "Four Waves of Feminism," *Pacific University Oregon.* October 25, 2015. https://www.pacificu.edu/magazine/four-waves-feminism.

Raphael, Rudly. "What Women Want: Love, Marriage and Dating." *Ebony,* March 7, 2019. https://www.ebony.com/life/ebony-attitudes/what-women-want-love-marriage-and-dating.

Read, Bridget. "It's Been 17 Years Since We First Heard About Mean Girls—Have We Learned Anything?" *Vogue,* April 23, 2018. https://www.vogue.com/article/did-we-learn-anything-from-mean-girls-musical-rosalind-wiseman-queen-bees-wannabees

Reilly, Eileen, Trish Hafford-Letchfield, and Nicky Lambert. "Women ageing solo in Ireland: An exploratory study of women's perspectives on relationship status and future care needs." *Qualitative Social Work,* 19, 1 (August 28, 2018): 75–92. https://doi.org/10.1177/1473325018796138.

"Read how IOA views aging in America." *Institute on Aging.* https://www.ioaging.org/aging-in-america.

"Relationship Status: Single—Dating Perceptions and Behaviors Among Generation X and Boomers." *AARP,* February 2019. https://doi.org/10.26419/res.00278.004.

Reti, Irene, and Sien, Shoney, editors. *Cats (and Their Dykes): An Anthology.* California: HerBooks, 1991.

Reuben, David. *Everything You Ever Wanted to Know About Sex* (*But Were Afraid to Ask).* First Edition. New York: McKay, 1969.

Richtel, Matt. "When an Ex-Spouse Returns as Caregiver." *New York Times,* May 19, 2005. https://www.nytimes.com/2005/05/19/fashion/thursdaystyles/when-an-exspouse-returns-as-caregiver.html.

Risman, Barbara J., Carissa Froyum, and William Scarborough, editors. *Handbook on the Sociology of Gender.* New York: Springer Publishers. 2018.

Robson, David. "The age you feel means more than your actual birthdate." *BBC Future,* July 19, 2018. https://www.bbc.com/future/article/20180712 -the-age-you-feel-means-more-than-your-actual-birthdate.

Rock, Lucy. "So now you're middle-aged? Pamela Druckerman can walk you through it." *The Guardian,* May 30, 2018. https://www.theguardian .com/society/2018/may/30/pamela-druckerman-there-are-no-grown-ups -midlife.

Rook, Karen S. "Gaps in Social Support Resources in Later Life: An Adaptational Challenge in Need of Further Research." *Journal of social and personal relationships,* 26, 1 (2009): 103–12. https://doi.org/10.1177/0265407509105525.

Rose, Suzanna M. "Enjoying the Returns: Women's Friendships After 50." In *Women Over 50,* edited by Varda Muhlbauer and Joan C. Chrisler, 112. Boston: Springer, 2007. https://doi.org/10.1007/978-0-387-46341-4_7.

Rosenbury, Laura A. "Friends with Benefits," Michigan Law Review 106, (2007): 189. http://scholarship.law.ufl.edu/facultypub/721.

Roseneil, Sasha. "Foregrounding Friendship: Feminist Pasts, Feminist Futures." In *Handbook of Gender and Women's Studies,* edited by Kathy Davis, Mary S. Evans, and Judith Lorber, 322–41. London: Sage Publications Ltd., 2006.

Rosenfeld, Michael J. "Are Tinder and Dating Apps Changing Dating and Mating in the U.S.?" *In Families and Technology,* edited by Jennifer Van Hook, Susan M. McHale, and Valarie King, 103–17. New York: Springer, 2018.

———. "Who Wants the Breakup? Gender and Breakup in Heterosexual Couples." In *Social Networks and the Life Course: Integrating the Development of Human Lives and Social Relational Networks, First Edition,* edited by Duane F. Alwin, Diane Felmlee, and Derek Kreager, 221–43. New York: Springer, 2018.

Rosenfeld, Michael J., and Reuben J. Thomas. "Searching for a Mate: The Rise of the Internet as a Social Intermediary." *American Sociological Review,* 77 (2012): 523–47. https://doi.org/10.1177/0003122412448050.

Rudman, Laurie A., and Stephanie A. Goodwin. "Gender differences in automatic in-group bias: Why do women like women more than men like men?" *Journal of Personality and Social Psychology,* 87, 4 (2004): 494–509. https://doi.org/10.1037/0022-3514.87.4.494.

Russell, Cristine. "Hair Today, Gray Tomorrow." *Washington Post,* October 8, 1989. https://www.washingtonpost.com/archive/lifestyle/well ness/1989/10/08/hair-today-gray-tomorrow/7abc2f13-e8b7-4f9b-a1d8 -08a88cc15668.

Saad, Lydia. "Children a Key Factor in Women's Desire to Work Outside the Home." *Gallup,* October 7, 2015. https://news.gallup.com/poll/186050/ children-key-factor-women-desire-work-outside-home.aspx.

Sabik, Natalie J. "Ageism and Body Esteem: Associations With Psychological Well-Being Among Late Middle-Aged African American and European American Women." *The Journals of Gerontology: Series B*, 70, 2 (2015): 189–99. https://doi.org/10.1093/geronb/gbt080.

Salisu, Margaret A., and Jagadisa-Devasri Dacus. "Living in a Paradox: How Older Single and Widowed Black Women Understand Their Sexuality." *Journal of Gerontological Social Work*, 64:3 (2021): 303–33. https://doi.org/10.1080/01634372.2020.1870603.

Sample, Ian. "Smiling Scots, worried Welsh and lazy Londoners: Survey maps regional personality types." *The Guardian*, March 24, 2015. https://www.theguardian.com/science/2015/mar/25/survey-maps-regional-personality-types.

Schaefer, Kayleen. *Text Me When You Get Home: The Evolution and Triumph of Modern Female Friendship*. New York: Dutton, 2018.

Schmidt, Susanne. *Midlife Crisis: The Feminist Origins of a Chauvinist Cliché*. Chicago: University of Chicago Press, 2020.

Schmitz, Rob. "China's Marriage Rate Plummets As Women Choose To Stay Single Longer," *NPR*, July 31, 2018. https://www.npr.org/2018/07/31/634048279/chinas-marriage-rate-plummets-as-women-choose-to-stay-single-longer.

Schreurs, Kathleen, Anabel Quan-Haase, and Kim Martin. "Problematizing the Digital Literacy Paradox in the Context of Older Adults' ICT Use: Aging, Media Discourse, and Self-Determination." *Canadian Journal of Communication* 42.2 (2017): 359–77.

Schumaker, Erin. "What we know about coronavirus' long-term effects." *ABC News*, April 17, 2020. https://abcnews.go.com/Health/coronavirus-long-term-effects/story?id=69811566.

Scribner, Sara. "Generation X gets really old: How do slackers have a midlife crisis?," *Salon*. August 11, 2013. https://www.salon.com/2013/08/11/generation_x_gets_really_old_how_do_slackers_have_a_midlife_crisis.

Settersten Jr., Richard A. "Some Things I Have Learned About Aging by Studying the Life Course." *Innovation in Aging*, 1, 2 (2017): igx014. https://doi.org/10.1093/geroni/igx014.

"Settling for less out of fear of being single," Correction to Spielmann et al. *Journal of personality and social psychology*. 115, 5 (2013) (2018): 804. https://doi.org/10.1037/pspp0000227.

Seymore, Teronda. "Practical Ways a Minimalist Lifestyle Frees Your Mind & Your Money." *XO Necole*, January 3, 2020. https://www.xonecole.com/minimalist-lifestyle-saves-money.

Shea, Danny. "Oprah Addresses Lesbian Rumors, Cries to Barbara Walters (VIDEO)," *HuffPost*, December 8, 2010. https://www.huffpost.com/entry/oprah-lesbian-rumors-cries-_n_793778.

Sheehy, Gail. *Passages: Predictable Crises of Adult Life*. First Edition. New York: E.P. Dutton & Co., 1976.

———. *Sex and the Seasoned Woman: Pursuing the Passionate Life.* New York: Ballantine Books, 2007.

Shpancer, Noam. "Feminine Foes: New Science Explores Female Competition." *Psychology Today,* January 26, 2014. https://www.psychology today.com/us/blog/insight-therapy/201401/feminine-foes-new-science -explores-female-competition.

"Singing spinster strikes a chord," *Associated Press,* April 17, 2009. https:// www.dailynews.com/2009/04/17/singing-spinster-strikes-a-chord.

"Singles in America: Match Releases Largest Study on U.S. Single Population for Eighth Year." February 1, 2018. https://www.prnewswire.com/ news-releases/singles-in-america-match-releases-largest-study-on-us -single-population-for-eighth-year-300591561.html.

Smith, Kristin. "Recessions Accelerate Trend of Wives as Breadwinners." *Carsey Institute,* 56 (2012). https://scholars.unh.edu/cgi/viewcontent .cgi?referer=https://www.google.com/&httpsredir=1&article=1180&cont ext=carsey.

Smith, Matthew Lee, H. H. Goltz, T. Coffey, and A. Boolani. "Sexually Transmitted Infection Knowledge among Older Adults: Psychometrics and Test-Retest Reliability." *International Journal of Environmental Research and Public Health* 17, 7 (2020): 2462. https://doi.org/10.3390/ijerph17072462.

Smith, Stacy L., Marc Choueiti, and Katherine Pieper. "Inclusion or Invisibility: Comprehensive Annenberg Report on Diversity in Entertainment." February 22, 2016. https://annenberg.usc.edu/sites/default/ files/2017/04/07/MDSCI_CARD_Report_FINAL_Exec_Summary.pdf.

Snow, Aurora. "Career-Minded Women Turn to Male Escorts for No-Strings Fun and (Maybe) Sex." *The Daily Beast,* January 3, 2015. https:// www.thedailybeast.com/career-minded-women-turn-to-male-escorts -for-no-strings-fun-and-maybe-sex.

Sobchack, Vivian. "Scary Women: Cinema, Surgery, and Special Effects" in *Figuring Age: Women, Bodies, Generations,* edited by Kathleen Woodward, 200–11. Indiana: Indiana University Press, 1999.

Solé, Elise. "More women over 50 are flaunting their bodies. And that's a good thing." *Yahoo Life,* December 20, 2019. https://www.yahoo.com/ now/more-women-over-50-are-flaunting-their-bodies-183709466.html.

Solomon, Alexandra H. *Taking Sexy Back: How to Own Your Sexuality and Create the Relationships You Want.* California: New Harbinger Publications, 2019.

Span, Paula. "Aging Without Children." *New York Times.* March 25, 2011. https://newoldage.blogs.nytimes.com/2011/03/25/aging-without -children.

Spector, Dina. "8 Scientifically Proven Reasons Life Is Better If You're Beautiful." *Insider,* June 12, 2013. https://www.businessinsider.com/studies -show-the-advantages-of-being-beautiful-2013-6.

Stainton, Hayley. "Female sex tourism. What does it mean and where does it happen?" *Tourism Teacher*, November 6, 2020. https://tourismteacher .com/female-sex-tourism.

Stanny, Barbara. "Money Coach and Author." Interview by Farnoosh Torabi. *So Money*, February 13, 2015. Audio, 31.25. https://podcast.farnoosh .tv/episode/barbara-stanny.

Stauffer, Rainesford. "Ageism Hurts All of Us, Even 'Young People.'" *Elle*, May 6, 2021. https://www.elle.com/life-love/a36290047/ageism-hurts-all -of-us-even-young-people.

Stepler, Renee. "Led by Baby Boomers, divorce rates climb for America's 50+ population." *Pew Research Center*, March 9, 2017. https://www.pew research.org/fact-tank/2017/03/09/led-by-baby-boomers-divorce-rates -climb-for-americas-50-population.

Stepler, Renee. "Smaller Share of Women Ages 65 and Older Are Living Alone," *Pew Research Center*, February 18, 2016. https://www.pewsocial trends.org/2016/02/18/smaller-share-of-women-ages-65-and-older-are -living-alone.

Stevens, Kara I. "4 Ways 'Strong Black Woman Syndrome' Keeps Us Poor." *Ebony*, December 11, 2019. https://www.ebony.com/career-finance/4 -ways-strongblack-woman-syndrome-keeps-us-poor-444.

Strauss, Judy R. "The Baby Boomers Meet Menopause: Fertility, Attractiveness, and Affective Response to the Menopausal Transition." *Sex Roles* 68 (2013): 77–90. https://doi.org/10.1007/s11199-011-0002-9.

Taylor, Shelley E., L. C. Klein, B. P. Lewis, T. L. Gruenewald, R. A. Gurung, and J. A. Updegraff. "Behaviorial Responses to Stress: Tend and Befriend, Not Fight or Flight." *Psychological Review* 107, 3 (2000): 41–429. https://doi .org/10.1037/0033-295x.107.3.411.

Taylor, Sonya Renee. *The Body Is Not an Apology Second Edition: The Power of Radical Self-Love*. California: Berrett-Koehler Publishers, 2021.

Tempesta, Erica. "Paulina Porizkova says she regrets allowing late husband Ric Ocasek to manage her money, saying it gave him total 'control' over her life—and made others view her as nothing more than 'the vapid wife of a rockstar.'" *The Daily Mail*, March 2, 2021. https://www.dailymail .co.uk/femail/article-9317873/Paulina-Porizkova-regrets-giving-late-hus band-Ric-Ocasek-control-money.html.

Tessier, Isabelle. "I Want To Be Single—But With You." *HuffPost*, July 17, 2015. https://www.huffpost.com/entry/i-to-be-single-but-with-you _b_7818158.

"That Age Old Question: How Attitudes to Ageing Affect Our Health and Wellbeing." *Royal Society for Public Health*, May 10, 2018. https://www .rsph.org.uk/static/uploaded/a01e3aa7-9356-40bc-99c81b14dd904a41.pdf.

Thayer, Colette. "Mirror/Mirror: AARP Survey of Women's Reflections on Beauty, Age, and Media." *AARP Research*, October 2018. https://doi .org/10.26419/res.00250.001.

Thomas, Holly N., M. Hamm, S. Borrero, R. Hess, and R. C. Thurston. "Body Image, Attractiveness, and Sexual Satisfaction Among Midlife Women: A Qualitative Study." *Journal of Women's Health* 28, 1 (2002): 100–106. https://doi.org/10.1089/jwh.2018.7107.

Tillotson, Kristin. "Many Women Come Out as Lesbians Later in Life." *Star Tribune (Minneapolis)*, January 21, 2010. https://www.postandcourier.com/features/many-women-come-out-as-lesbians-later-in-life/article_6be6af57-e9ee-5f44-a4bc-9b17dba0ed59.html.

Torabi, Farnoosh. "I've been writing about money for 15 years, and here are the 9 best pieces of financial advice I can give you." *Insider*, October 7, 2015. https://www.businessinsider.com/personal-finance/best-money-advice-farnoosh-torabi-2015-10#-2.

———. "Wives: Stop Leaving Money Management to Your Spouse." *Bloomberg*, November 14, 2020. https://www.bloomberg.com/opinion/articles/2020-11-14/personal-finance-advice-for-women-avoiding-money-in-marriage.

Travis, Cheryl Brown, and C. P. Yeager. "Sexual Selection, Parental Investment, and Sexism." *Journal of Social Issues*, 47 (1991): 117–29. https://doi.org/10.1111/j.1540-4560.1991.tb01826.x.

Tree, Jennifer M. Jabson, Joanne G. Patterson, Daniel P. Beavers, and Deborah J. Bowen. "What Is Successful Aging in Lesbian and Bisexual Women? Application of the Aging-Well Model." *The Journals of Gerontology: Series B* (2020): gbaa130. https://doi.org/10.1093/geronb/gbaa130.

Tugend, Alina. "When Only One Spouse Retires." *Kiplinger*, November 20, 2020. https://www.kiplinger.com/retirement/601791/when-only-one-spouse-retires.

UBS. "Own Your Worth 2021: Building bridges, breaking barriers." May 6, 2021. http://www.static-ubs.com/content/dam/assets/wma/us/documents/own-your-worth-building-bridges-Q221-us-en.pdf.

———. "New UBS report reveals that joint financial participation is the key to gender equality." July 6, 2020. https://www.ubs.com/global/en/media/display-page-ndp/en-20200706-key-to-gender-equality.html.

University at Buffalo. "Age discrimination laws don't protect older women as they do older men," June 18, 2020, *ScienceDaily*. www.sciencedaily.com/releases/2020/06/200618120157.htm.

University of Delaware. "Views of ideal female appearance in China are changing." *Phys.org*, November 28, 2018. https://phys.org/news/2018-11-views-ideal-female-china.html.

University of Miami. "Women's pain not taken as seriously as men's pain: A new study suggests that when men and women express the same amount of pain, women's pain is considered less intense based on gender stereotypes." *ScienceDaily*. www.sciencedaily.com/releases/2021/04/210406164124.htm.

U.S. Census Bureau. "Unmarried and Single Americans Week: Sept. 17–23, 2017." August 14, 2017. https://www.census.gov/newsroom/facts-for -features/2017/single-americans-week.html.

———. "Historical Marital Status Tables." December 2020. https://www .census.gov/data/tables/time-series/demo/families/marital.html.

———. "Number, Timing, and Duration of Marriages and Divorces: 2009," May 2011. https://www.census.gov/prod/2011pubs/p70-125.pdf.

Vale, Michael T., Toni L. Bisconti, and Jennifer F. Sublett. "Benevolent ageism: Attitudes of overaccommodative behavior toward older women." *The Journal of Social Psychology*, 160, 5, (2020): 548–58. DOI: 10.1080/00224545.2019.1695567.

Vandenakker, Carol B., and Dorothea D. Glass. "Menopause and aging with disability." *Physical medicine and rehabilitation clinics of North America*, 12, 1 (2001): 133–51. https://doi.org/10.1016/S1047-9651(18)30087-1.

Van den Hoonaard, Deborah. "Attitudes of older widows and widowers in New Brunswick, Canada toward new partnerships." *Ageing International*, 27, 4 (2002): 79–92. https://doi.org/10.1007/s12126-002-1016-y.

Van Meter, Jonathan. "How Kris Jenner Is Taking the Kardashian-Jenner Empire to Hulu and Beyond." *Wall Street Journal Magazine*, March 23, 2021. https://www.wsj.com/articles/kris-jenner-interview-kardashian-kim -kanye-chrissy-11616502549.

Velez, Adriana. "Menopause Is Different for Women of Color." *EndocrineWeb*, March 10, 2021. https://www.endocrineweb.com/menopause -different-women-color.

Veresiu, Ela. "The #advancedstyle movement celebrates and empowers stylish older women." *The Conversation*, April 19, 2021. https://thecon versation.com/the-advancedstyle-movement-celebrates-and-empowers -stylish-older-women-157952.

Wade, Lisa. "Women are less happy than men in marriage, so why does the media insist otherwise?" *Sociological Images*, December 27, 2016. https:// thesocietypages.org/socimages/2016/12/27/women-are-less-happy-than -men-in-marriage-so-why-does-the-media-insist-otherwise.

Walker, Alicia. *Secret Life of the Cheating Wife: Power, Pragmatism, and Pleasure in Women's Infidelity*. Maryland: Lexington Books, 2017.

"Wage Gap May Help Explain Why More Women Are Anxious and Depressed Than Men." *Columbia Mailman School of Health*, January 5, 2016. https://www.publichealth.columbia.edu/public-health-now/news/wage -gap-may-help-explain-why-more-women-are-anxious-and-depressed-men.

Watson, Wendy K., and Charlie Stelle. "Dating for older women: Experiences and meanings of dating in later life." *Journal of Women & Aging*, 23, 3 (2011): 263–75. https://doi.org/10.1080/08952841.2011.587732.

Waxman, Barbara. "Celebrate Life's Newest Stage: Middlescence." *Forbes*. August 29, 2016. https://www.forbes.com/sites/nextavenue/2016/08/29/ celebrate-lifes-newest-stage-middlescence.

Weiner, Jennifer. "I Feel Personally Judged by J. Lo's Body," *New York Times*, February 4, 2020. https://www.nytimes.com/2020/02/04/opinion/jlo-superbowl-performance.html.

Weinstock, Jacqueline S. "Lesbian friendships at midlife: Patterns and possibilities for the 21st century." *Journal of Gay & Lesbian Social Services*, 11 (2000): 1–32. doi: 10.1300/j041v11n02_01.

Weinstock, Jacqueline S., and Esther D. Rothblum. "Just friends: The role of friendship in lesbians' lives." *Journal of Lesbian Studies*, 22:1 (2018), 1–3. doi:10.1080/10894160.2017.1326762.

West, Keon. "Naked and Unashamed: Investigations and Applications of the Effects of Naturist Activities on Body Image, Self-Esteem, and Life Satisfaction." *Journal of Happiness Studies* 19 (2018): 677–97. https://doi.org/10.1007/s10902-017-9846-1.

Weston, Kath. *Families We Choose: Lesbians, Gays, Kinship (Between Men–between Women)*. New York: Columbia University Press, May 1, 1991.

Wilson-Beattie, Robin. "Bodies in Transition." *Pulp*, December 10, 2019. https://medium.com/pulpmag/bodies-in-transition-34020653f782.

Wiley, Clare. "Relationship Anarchy Takes the Judgment Out of Love." *Medium*, August 6, 2015. https://medium.com/@Clare_Wiley/relationship-anarchy-takes-the-judgment-out-of-love-1c7838e97d3.

Williams, Mary Elizabeth. "'Unwell Women' author Elinor Cleghorn: Women's pain 'isn't taken seriously' by doctors." *Salon*, June 8, 2021. https://www.salon.com/2021/06/08/unwell-women-author-elinor-cleghorn-womens-pain-isnt-taken-seriously-by-doctors.

Winfrey, Oprah. "Oprah Explains Why She and Gayle King "Will Always be in Each Other's Corner." *Oprah Daily*, August 7, 2019. https://www.oprahdaily.com/life/a28323160/oprah-gayle-friendship-memories.

Wischhover, Cheryl. "The fall of 'anti-aging' skin care." *Vox*, September 11, 2018. https://www.vox.com/the-goods/2018/9/11/17840984/skin-care-anti-aging-drunk-elephant.

Wiseman, Rosalind. "Dealing With Grown-Up 'Mean Girls.'" *New York Times*, December 5, 2019. https://www.nytimes.com/2019/12/05/well/family/dealing-with-grown-up-mean-girls.html.

Wolf, Naomi. *The Beauty Myth: How Images of Beauty Are Used Against Women*. Reprint Edition. New York: Harper Perennial, 2002.

"Women & Financial Wellness: Beyond the Bottom Line." Merrill Lynch and Age Wave, 2019. https://www.bofaml.com/content/dam/boamlimages/documents/articles/ID18_0244/ml_womens_study.pdf.

"Women More Likely Than Men to Initiate Divorces, But Not Non-Marital Breakups." *American Sociological Association*. August 22, 2015. https://www.asanet.org/press-center/press-releases/women-more-likely-men-initiate-divorces-not-non-marital-breakups.

The Woody Allen Pages, "Everything You Always Wanted to Know About Sex* (*But Were Afraid to Ask)." Accessed April 27, 2021. http://www

.woodyallenpages.com/films/everything-you-always-wanted-to-know
-about-sex-but-were-afraid-to-ask.

Yarrow, Andrew L. "I spoke to hundreds of American men who still can't find work." *Vox*, September 17, 2018. https://www.vox.com/first-person /2018/9/15/17859134/recession-financial-crisis-2018-men.

Yavorsky, Jill, and Janette Dill. "Unemployment and men's entrance into female-dominated jobs." *Social Science Research* 85 (2020): 102373. doi:10.1016/j.ssresearch.2019.102373.

You, Tracy. "The last foot-binding survivors: Chinese grandmothers uncover their deformed 'lotus feet'—a symbol of beauty less than a century ago." *The Daily Mail*, February 27, 2018. https://www.dailymail.co.uk/ news/article-5425801/Last-foot-binding-survivors-captured-beautiful -photos.html.

Yu, Rebecca P., Nicole B. Ellison, Ryan J. McCammon, and Kenneth M. Langa. "Mapping the Two Levels of Digital Divide: Internet Access and Social Network Site Adoption among Older Adults in the USA." *Information, Communication & Society*, 19, 10 (2016): 1445–64. https://doi.org/10.10 80/1369118X.2015.1109695.

Zomorodi, Manoush. "A Self-Indulgent Ode to Old Lady Hair." *Human Parts*, November 17, 2020. https://humanparts.medium.com/old-lady -hair-a67eb312ae8c.

Zetlin, Minda. "Will Staying Home Lead to More Divorces? 45 Percent of Millennials and Gen-Z Say Yes." *Inc.*, April 17, 2020. https://www.inc .com/minda-zetlin/divorce-rates-coronavirus-relationships-strain-social -distancing.html.

Zhang, Zhenmei, and Mark D. Hayward. "Childlessness and the Psychological Well-Being of Older Persons." *The Journals of Gerontology: Series B*, 56, 5, 1 (September 2001): S311–S320. https://doi.org/10.1093/ geronb/56.5.S311.

Ziegler, Ali, Jes L. Matsick, Amy C. Moors, Jennifer Rubin, and Terri Conley. "Does monogamy harm women? Deconstructing monogamy with a feminist lens." [Special Issue on Polyamory]. *Journal für Psychologie*, 22, 1 (2014): 1–18. https://www.journal-fuer-psychologie.de/index.php/jfp/ article/view/323/354.

Index

Acevedo, Beatriz, 148
"advanced style" movement, 93
The Afrominimalist's Guide to Living with Less (Platt), 146
Ageing Well Without Children, United Kingdom, 23
ageism: finance ramifications of, 133; health ramifications of, 123; older women and benevolent, 116; Segal on, 155–56; women and, 118, 154
"Ageism Can Be Hazardous to Women's Health" (Chrisler), 116
"agelessness," x, 3
aging, 106–8, 152–54; African "Sawubona" greeting and, 24; becoming narratives in, 5; deciding for ourselves in, 6; Donizzetti on, 154; future self realistic version in, 4, 9, 157; Generation X and ageist narratives in, 5–6; gerontologists ideas on, 4; honest conversations about, 155; intentionality in, 4; mid-sixties and, 124–25; new narratives creation about, 155, 156; no right way in, 8; old narratives danger in, 14–15; queer and crip theories applied to, 9; reflection questions about,

129; romantic love beliefs and, 71–72; Sobchack on, 4–5; society messages about, 3, 4; Stauffer on, 156; Waldman on, 20–21
aging successfully: as best we can, 128; concept of, 125; coronavirus pandemic and, 128; cultural narratives and, 126; Gen Xers and Millennials expectations in, 128; Holstein on, 125–26; lesbian and bisexual women impact of, 127; as lifelong process, 126; mandates for, 125; men and women impact of, 126; our fault in, 125; physical or cognitive disabilities and, 127; reflection questions about, 129; SMW and, 127; Strong Black Woman stereotype in, 126–27; woman's body sexualizing in, 126; women with disabilities and, 127–29
Allen, Amelia, 92
Allen, Eugenie, 137
Allen, Neal, 66–67
The All-Or-Nothing Marriage (Finkel), 100
Allure magazine, "anti-aging" term use ban of, 77
"amatonormativity," 50, 51, 103
Angier, Natalie, 35

227

in, 50; mother heart-to-heart talk
about marriage and, 57–58; older
lesbians challenges in, 70; older
men and younger women in, 67;
older women and, 67–68; older
women and romantic partners
in, 52–53; online and dating apps
in, 70–71; open marriage and,
57; pandemic impact on, 61; Pell,
on love late in life, 69; reflection
questions about, 72; romantic
love beliefs and, 71–72; romantic
notions and society-approved
script of, 53–54; Sandberg and
Bernthal in, 66; "self-partnered"
and, 49–50, 53; society and
different messages about, 50;
spouse and living apart in,
58; subordination and, 58;
Taylor-Johnson, A., and Taylor-
Johnson, S., age gap in, 67;
true partnership in, 58; Watson
on anxiety and, 49–50; what
do I want question in, 53–54;
widowhood average age and, 51;
women stereotypes and societal
pressure about, 52; women with
disabilities challenges in, 70
Love and Trouble (Dederer), 38
Love Warrior (Doyle), 43
Lövgren, Karin, 63

MacArthur Foundation Study of
Aging in America, 125
Maciel, Michelle, 30, 34
Macron, Emmanuel, 67
Maestas, Nicole, 142
Make Love, Not Porn, 32
Margolies, Lynn, 96
marriage. *See* love and marriage
Martin, Wednesday, 35
Match.com, 35, 68
Mattern, Susan, 16
McClanahan, Rue, 82, 97

McCrory, Helen, 88–89
McDormand, Frances, 80, 88, 152,
154
McGrath, Laura, 24
McRuer, Robert, 22, 23
Mead, Margaret, 15
Mead, Rebecca, 138
Mean Girls, 95
men, 29–30, 86, 133, 140, 151–52;
aging successfully impact on,
126; health-care system and
pain intensity of, 123; love and
marriage and, 67; menopause
study and understanding
of, 121–22; as undermining
friendship cause, 100; women
pay difference and, 132, 143;
women's sexuality and younger,
32
menopause, 30, 115, 118; article
headlines about, 119; average
age for, 119; Black and Latina
women and, 120; childless and
childfree women and, 120;
disabled women and, 120; as
disease, 16; as end of useful life
mark, 14; Gen X women and,
119; "grandmother hypothesis"
of, 16; health and stereotypes
in, 10; health impact of, 119;
hormonal changes and other
health risks of, 119; horror stories
of, 1; knowledge gap about,
120; marriage and reproduction
delay impact on, 19; Mead,
M., on "postmenopausal
zest," 15; medicalization and
pathologizing of, 16; men
study and understanding
about, 121–22; mind shift in,
1–2; reflection questions about,
129; romantic partners and,
120; as "second youth," 16;
shame and stigma about, 121;

Walsh, Wendy, 86
Wambach, Abby, 43
Warren, Elizabeth, 86
Watson, Emma, 49–50, 72
Waxman, Barbara, 18
WealthiHer, 149
Weiner, Jennifer, 85
Weinstock, Jacqueline S., 103
Weston, Kath, 97
What Happy Women Do (Kudak), 111
When Harry Met Sally, 29
White, Betty, 82
Why We Can't Sleep (Calhoun), 5, 39
Williamson, Marianne, 86
Wilson-Beattie, Robin, 37, 70
Winfrey, Oprah, 91, 98–99, 100
Wiseman, Rosalind, 95
Wolf, Naomi, 81, 94
women: age denial of, 117; ageism
  and, 118, 154; ageist attitudes
  change of, 154; aging feelings
  and awareness of, 152; aging
  honest conversations of, 155;
  childfree rise in, 64; childless
  "die-alone" scenario of, 65;
  without children, 23; disability
  stats on, 22; divorce and, 55–56;
  "do as I say, not as I do" and,
  153; early ageism of, 153;
  financial success knowledge
  of, 152; as "functionally
  unnecessary," 13–14; "The future
  is female" slogan and, 156; as
  ignored and undermined and
  overlooked, 151; invisibility
  experiences of, 19; invisibility
  meaning to, 12; Kendrick on
  being single, 64–65; male-
  dominated environment buy
  in of, 151–52; marginalized
  challenges of, 21; narrative
  changing of, 152–53; Ojewumi
  on black women and disability,
  22; potential development of,

151; questioning and sorting
  aging feelings and, 152;
  reproductive age focus on, 12;
  self-acceptance idea for, 153;
  societal expectations of, 20;
  teenage girls and "premature
  aging" trend in, 153–54. *See also*
  specific topics
women's sexuality, 126; affairs
  and, 41–42; asexual menopausal
  woman stereotype in, 30;
  Boomers and sexual revolution
  in, 36; Brooks, K., on, 39;
  Calhoun on, 39; compromise and
  restraint multiple layers in, 35;
  consensual non-monogamy in,
  41; Dederer on, 38–39; desired
  being challenge in, 40; disabled
  women and, 37; divorce and, 38;
  doctors and sex topic in, 45; ebb
  and flow of desire in, 28; Eve's
  mother's orgasm story and,
  27–28; expansive possibilities
  in, 44; FWB embracing in, 31;
  Gallop on younger men and
  older women, 32; "geriatric
  sexuality breakdown syndrome"
  message in, 34; *Good Luck to
  You, Leo Grande* plotline and,
  30–31; Gunter on libido issue
  in, 45; health and medication
  impacting, 33–34; Jong on, 27;
  late-life same-sex attraction in,
  43–44; "lesbian bed death" and,
  28, 44; libido loss and, 29; life
  circumstances and, 40; Little
  League game conversation
  about, 37–38; male erectile
  dysfunction and, 29, 30; Murray
  on sexual desire, 29–30; "new
  aging" movement discourse and,
  44–45; new lovers and libido
  boost in, 38; older Black women
  and, 34–35; older Mexican-

American women and, 45; older
people and sex societal belief
in, 33; older single women
stereotypes in, 32; older women
and interest in, 27, 28, 30, 32–33;
one-sided sexual experiences
in, 31; open marriages in, 42;
outdated beliefs about, 28;
passion and pleasure and
intimacy desire in, 28–29; paying
for sex option and study in,
31; physical and psychological
health in, 35; polyamory
and, 41; positive attitude in,
34; questionable beliefs and
assumptions in, 35–36; reflection
questions about, 47; sex and
creativity in, 36; "sex tourism"
and, 31; sexual awakening in,
42–43; sexual satisfaction outside

of marriage and, 29, 39–40;
sexual self-expression limiting
in, 36; "Singles in America"
survey of, 35; society and aging
body in, 34; speaking up about,
46; standard evolutionary
psychology troupe on, 40;
strong and healthy images in,
35; Thomas, H., on, 46; vaginal
changes and, 33; Western culture
overemphasis on sex and, 36;
When Harry Met Sally scene and,
29; Wilson-Beattie on, 37
Woodard, Kirsty, 23
Woolf, Virginia, 98

Yeah, No. Not Happening (Karbo), 81

Ziegler, Ali, 41
Zomorodi, Manoush, 81

About the Author

Vicki Larson is a longtime award-winning journalist and co-author of *The New I Do: Reshaping Marriage for Skeptics, Realists and Rebels*. The lifestyles editor, columnist, and writer at the *Marin Independent Journal*, Larson's writing can also be found in the *New York Times*, the *Washington Post, The Guardian, Aeon, Medium,* and *HuffPost* among other places. Larson has also been a guest on several radio and television shows, including Minnesota Public Radio, the BBC, Canada's *The Morning Show* and *The Social*, as well as podcasts, including *The Femsplainers* and *Solo: The Single Person's Guide to a Remarkable Life*. She is the mother of two young men and lives in the San Francisco Bay Area.